TABLE OF CONTENTS

Purpose and Introduction 7

Using This Guide 9

The Caregivers Guide to Taking Care Of Loved Ones & Themselves 13

    10 Tips to Make Your New Role Easier 13

A Caregiver's Feelings 16

    Your Own Needs 17

    Long Distance Care 19

    Caregiver Stress 20

    5 Things Not to Say to Someone with a Chronic Illness 21

Overall, It Takes Time 23

Chronic Kidney Disease Overview 25

    The workings of the kidney 25

    Symptoms and risk factors of kidney disease 26

    Progression and prevalence of disease 28

    Chronic Kidney Disease (CKD) 30

Foreword 35

    Dear Reader, ... 35

Mrs. Murray's Caregivers 37

    Caregivers and caregiving costs 37

    Caring for my mother with CKD 38

    The professional caregiver 40

Mrs. Murray's Condition Worsens 43

    How it started and where it is now 43

    Lifestyle adaptations for someone with CKD 44

    Caring for a caregiver 46

    Mrs. Murray's options 48

Mrs. Murray's Depression	51
Letting Janice go	51
Mrs. Murray's depression	53
Transplant Surgery and Dialysis	59
We first examined transplant surgery	59
Home Hemodialysis (HHD)	61
I Have Become Mom's Caregiver	65
The Caregiver's Predicament	65
Parting words	68
Dear Reader	71
Epilogue	73
Introduction to Aromatherapy	77
What is Aromatherapy?	78
What are Essential Oils?	78
Massage	82
Homeopathic doses	85
Holistic Healing	89
The whole	89
The aura and chakras	89
The 7 main chakras are:	91
Emotional connections with kidneys and sacral chakra	93
Oils for the kidneys	95
Oils which should be avoided in Chronic Kidney Disease are:	99
Helping the physical symptoms brought on by chronic kidney disease	101
Oils for the emotions	101
Oils for the caregiver	103
Contraindications and safety data	103
Buying essential oils	105

- Correct labeling 105
- Storing essential oils 106

Bibliography 109

An Overview 113

Understanding Reflexology Treatment 115
- Defining Reflexology 115
- How it Works 115

How Effective is Reflexology for Kidney Failure 119

The Reflexology Area 121
- Structure of the Feet and Hands 121
- Crucial Zones 121

Things to Consider Before Starting Reflexology 123

Implementing Reflexology Treatment 125
- Duration and Frequency of Reflexology 125
- Massage Techniques 126

Parting Words 131

Introduction 135

The Cranial Rhythm 137
- Somato Emotional Release 140

CranioSacral Therapy and Kidney Disease 141
- What conditions can CST address that might be valuable for CKD? 141

The Treatment Process 145
- How the treatment process works 145

CranioSacral Therapists 149
- Certification programs 149

Simple Techniques to Try at Home 153

Conclusion 158

Worksheets Section 159

Purpose and Introduction

What I have found through the emails and requests of my readers is that it is difficult to find information about chronic kidney disease and the lifestyle that is actionable. I want you to know that is what I intend to provide in all my books.

I wrote this guide with you in mind: the person with kidney problems who does not know where to start or can't seem to get the answers that you need from other sources. This guide will provide information that is applicable to a kidney disease lifestyle.

Who am I? I am a registered dietitian in the USA who has been working with kidney patients for my entire 15 + years of experience.

<u>My goals are simple</u> – to give some answers and to create an understanding of what is typical. I will take you through the different parts of being a caregiver to the person with kidney disease. It will not necessarily be what happens in your case, as everyone is an individual. I may simplify things in an effort to write them so that I feel you can learn the most from the information. This may mean that I don't say the exact things that your doctor would say. If you don't understand, please ask your doctor.

I want you to know, I am not a medical doctor and I am not aware of your particular condition. Information in this book is current as of publication, but may or may not have changed. This book is not meant to substitute for medical treatment for you, your friends, your caregivers, or your family members. You should not base treatment decisions solely on what is contained in this book. Develop your treatment plan with your doctors, nurses and the other medical professionals on your team. I recommend that you double-check any information with your medical team to verify if it applies to you.

In other words, I am not responsible for your medical care. I am providing this book for information and entertainment purposes, not medical diagnoses. Please consult with your doctor about any questions that you have about your particular case.

© 2017 Renal Diet Headquarters, www.renaldiethq.com , All Rights Reserved. No reproduction without author's written permission

Using This Guide

1. Review the overview for caregivers in section 1. This is designed to orient you to the guide and start you on the right foot.
2. If you need information about Chronic Kidney Disease, read the overview in section 2. This gives you a general glance about what the disease is and how it will progress for most people.
3. Read Mrs. Murray's story. It's a quick read looking at the emotions of caregivers and using home health care if you can. It also looks at the family's decisions to start taking on the care themselves and moving Mrs. Murray to the dialysis stage of CKD.
4. If you are interested in doing some alternative medicine care for your loved one, read the aromatherapy, reflexology, and craniosacral therapy chapters. They are helpful for both yourself and the loved one. You can share them with your physician if they have questions, and discuss using any sort of complementary medicine with them prior to starting.
5. Make copies of the included worksheets to use to start tracking care for your loved one. Use the information in your doctor's visits and if you have any other providers to be consistent across all areas. Those are located in the last section of the book and through the link indicated in that section to find them online and printable copies to download.
6. Send any feedback about the book or errors to renaldiethq@gmail.com

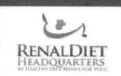

OVERVIEW OF CHRONIC KIDNEY DISEASE FOR CAREGIVERS

Learn More About Renal Disease

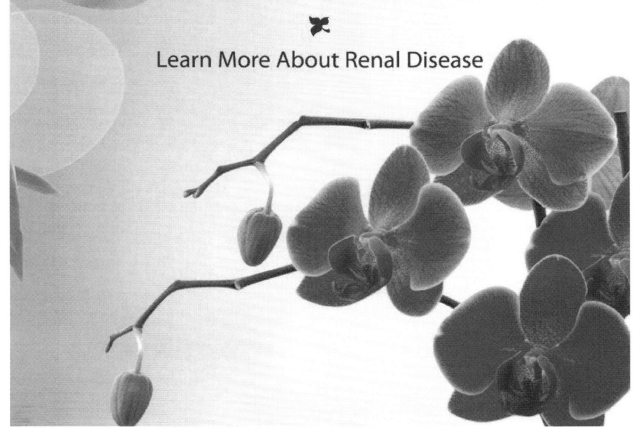

The Caregivers Guide to Taking Care Of Loved Ones & Themselves

Most of the attention is given to the person who has been diagnosed with the chronic illness. They, after all, are the ones who suffer the physical and emotional effects of the illness the most. However, it's important not to overlook their caregivers. Family members and friends can still be affected. In fact, caregivers often suffer their own emotional distress and have few outlets in which to address them.

As a caregiver, you may face many new responsibilities you didn't have to deal with before. Some of these might feel overwhelming. You may feel isolated and alone. There will be other times, when care giving to your loved might feel rewarding. Luckily, there are things you can do to make the process easier for both of you.

There are a few different kinds of caregiver situations. For instance, you might be caring for a spouse or you could be responsible for administering care to a parent or perhaps your child. No matter what your circumstance is, your new role is going to take some getting used to. It also depends on the type of care you are giving – is your family member going to be living with you, or going to an adult living center where the level of care is adjusted based on their condition? Assisted living or nursing center? When you know what these mean, you can make better decisions. If you are older and caring for your spouse, do you have an option to move closer to a family member so they could help?

Family caregivers are almost never trained for the responsibilities with which they are suddenly faced. Most caregivers are not healthcare providers themselves nor ever anticipated the situation that they suddenly find themselves in. Of course, as a caregiver, you still want to provide the best care you can to your loved one.

10 Tips to Make Your New Role Easier

1. **Learn as much as you can about your loved one's medical condition**. Knowledge is power and you'll feel far less overwhelmed when you understand what is going on in their bodies and how you can manage their needs. In this guide, we spend time talking about what the disease is and how you can expect it to progress. Your loved one's may not follow the exact same path, but it will have some similarities. Having a path and

understanding where you are going helps with controlling the fear and apprehension you might be feeling.

2. **Take breaks**. You must get out from time to time and do things outside of the illness. You didn't choose the role that you are now in and sometimes you need a mental health break in order to see to your own needs. This could be taking a walk around the neighborhood or going out with friends. Make sure you also take some caregiver vacations – times when you allow others to do the work you do everyday for your loved one and give yourself a chance to relax. Being the only caregiver is extremely stressful, and considering this is a 24 hour a day job – ask other family members to step in at regular intervals or find out if you can utilize some home health care that will come in and do some of the more difficult tasks with bathing and wound care if needed.

3. **Find support**. See if you can connect with other caregivers. Knowing that you are not alone is comforting. Not only can it be helpful to talk to others so that you can gain support, you might find that giving support to others is also helpful. A caregiver group may be available as part of your doctor's office or may be through a local hospital. Search them out. Find out if a local chapter of a kidney disease support group is in your area – contact www.kidney.org or www.aakp.org

4. **Be an advocate for your loved one**. Never ignore what your loved one's doctors are telling them. But, you spend more time with them on a daily basis, and you're closer to the situation. If you feel the need for more information or changes to care, speak up. Use the worksheets included in this guide to track your loved one's care that you are giving and to keep track of what you need to know. Learning the patterns of what is happening is very helpful to your doctor so you can give them as much information as possible about things that happen. Saying "it happens every day at 11 am" is better than "I think it happens most days but I am not sure when". Being able to quantify with time and frequency allows them to eliminate some issues and brings to light others.

5. **Find a stress outlet**. Learn to journal, blog, crochet, or whatever it is you need to de-stress. Caring for someone else is time consuming and takes a lot

of emotional energy. Try your best to find an outlet that will allow you to work off any frustration or stress. You will have time during doctor appointments waiting to be called in, or even when your loved one may be napping. Keep doing some things for yourself to reduce the stress you are feeling.

6. **Take care of yourself**. You still have your own health issues to worry about, too. Don't forget that lack of sleep, lack of exercise, and poor diet can have mental and physical effects on your body just as it does on your loved one. Watch for signs of depression and ensure you don't let yourself get down in the dumps. Being realistic is important, and if your loved one's health is worsening you need to accept that. But being sad about it won't change the direction they are going – acting according to their doctor's recommendations will help.

7. **Help, but don't do everything for them**. You are there to help them when necessary. You should try to encourage your loved one's independence. Through their independence they can gain confidence and self-assurance. Many times they let you do things because you are there, but continually doing things for them can remove their independence and lead to more reliance on you. Ask them if they are comfortable doing the task, stand by ready to help, but give them the chance to try if you can.

8. **Be realistic**. You might feel like a superhero sometimes, but you're not one. Learn your limits and stick to them. Don't spread yourself too thin. If you have a hard time driving a lot or in certain times of the day, ask for help. Make appointments all on one day instead of throughout the week so you can have some sanity. Ask for what you need, and most of the time people will be willing to adjust.

9. **Ask for help**. Other family members and friends are probably more than happy to pitch in and help on occasion. Most people are just standing by, waiting for someone to tell them what they need. Don't be afraid to use other resources. The truth is, they do not know how difficult of a time you are having until you tell them. They assume you are fine. So, ask if you need a little help, or a break, and see if you can use some local resources – like a Senior Center or Meals on Wheels.

10. **Keep a support network**. It's easy to lose yourself in the needs of your loved one. Keep in touch, however, with your own friends and other family members. Don't pretend like your feelings don't matter – they do. You are better able to take care of your loved one when you are relaxed and coping well. Finding someone to relate your stress and frustrations to that is NOT the person you are caring for is very important. You can "vent" and get it out and many times that will help you think about what you need to do to fix your issue. Or maybe your issue was just needing to talk.

A Caregiver's Feelings

Caregiving can set off lots of difficult emotions. Some of these can be guilt-inducing, especially when it comes to feeling angry and resentful. Other times, you might feel helpless and even scared. Rather than hiding or avoiding your feelings, try to acknowledge and accept what you're feeling, even the bad stuff. Your feelings don't mean that you don't love your loved one. You're only human and it's normal to experience a range of emotions in the face of new challenges. Also understand, however, that when you do feel things like anger and resentment that you're feeling them towards the illness and not the actual person.

Some feelings you might feel yourself facing include:

- Anger
- Worry
- Anxiety
- Stress
- Resentment
- Guilt
- Grief
- Frustration
- Depression
- Fear
- Helplessness

Some of these feelings might feel irrational. You might worry about the new responsibilities and how you will handle them. You might be afraid of what will happen to your loved one, should they start deteriorating quickly. You might even feel resentful towards other people in your life that you feel should also be sharing your burden. Lastly, it's normal to feel jealous of others who don't share the same responsibilities as you do.

It can still be upsetting to feel the way you do, even when you have a good grasp as to why you're feeling certain feelings. Finding a healthy environment in which to deal with these feelings is important. Recognizing them and then sharing with a trusted support individual, either a doctor or close friend, can help you learn to process the feelings and to move past them.

Your Own Needs

It's easy to forget your own needs when you're caring for someone else, but you shouldn't. Your own physical, mental, and even social needs should not be ignored. After all, you also deserve to experience a high quality of life.

If you are a spouse, you might be expected to have some responsibilities that a child would not have. You also might be suffering from some chronic illness issues of your own. If you are trying to maintain a household and manage the bills for a chronic illness that can be overwhelming. That said, you may not want to live with your children or move to an assisted living facility. Hard choices have to be made, but take your own feelings into account as you will have to live with the outcomes.

One important thing about moving is that you lose connection with people you have been around naturally for a long time. If you have raised children in a neighborhood, to suddenly move out of that area can result in isolation if you don't find ways to reconnect or connect with new people.

As a child caring for a parent, you might have a family of your own to care for too. Their lives will be affected, and you should try to involve your family in as much of the process as possible. Grandma or Grandpa coming to live with you sounds like a good solution, but it might affect you at meal times, doing laundry, and other routines you have. Taking on responsibility might mean reducing hours or quitting your job. With the need to take the member of your family on medical appointments or even just be available to care for them, many employers won't be able to accommodate your needs.

Emotional needs

- **Learn stress relieving techniques so that when you become stressed and anxious your mental health isn't suffering**.

- Find a way to communicate your feelings. This can be in the form of journaling, talking to a friend, or within the confines of a support group.

- Find ways to enjoy the things that you love. You might not be able to do them as often as you'd like, but it's important to keep doing them.

- Find a doctor and seek care if things become too hard and stressful.

- Talk to your patient's caregiver about additional support options such as home health

- Understand the medical benefits the insurance you have provides. What sort of medicine can be ordered in generic or do you have access to home health? Call the company and ask if you need to.

Social needs

- See and connect with other people in person. Make an effort to maintain a social life. It's important for the caregiver not to feel isolated and lonely.

- Get out of the house when you can. Go for a walk, go to the movies, or just go out to eat from time to time.

- Continue to enjoy your hobbies and your work, if you're still able to.

- Find a social network around you. Consider joining a church, a group, or a club that meets regularly.

Physical needs

- **Exercise.** Regular physical activity can help keep your mind and body healthy. Physical activity is important for maintaining your physical health but can also help stave off depression and anxiety.

- **Eat well.** Lack of daily vitamins and minerals can wreck havoc on your health. Maintaining your physical health is important for your energy and emotional health.

- **Make healthy decisions.** Learn healthy outlets for managing your stress, because when you're care giving it's easy to become overwhelmed. If it does become too much, then talk to your doctor about prescriptions or counseling that might help you manage signs of depression.

- **Rest.** Proper sleep is important to your body. Lack of sleep can make you open for infections. It can also increase weight gain and cut off your supply of energy. Without the right amount of sleep, your body is unable to renew itself. This might leave you feeling tired and irritable.

Long Distance Care

Sometimes you might find yourself as the caregiver for a loved one who doesn't live within a close proximity. Managing their care from a distance can increase feelings of guilt and anxiety. There might be other feelings involved as well. To ease the burden of responsibility, consider following the steps below to help ensure your loved one is safe and provided for.

- **Create an alarm.** Since the distance between you and your loved one is great, you might to invest in an electronic alarm system. You can't get to them in time if something happens but at least you will know that they can call for help.
- **Be a part of medical appointments.** Schedule any medical appointments at a time when you can attend them. If you can, schedule them all within the same timeframe to make it easier. Have your loved one sign a privacy release (or advance directive) so that you can talk to their doctors on their behalf if needed. An advance directive is a legal document that lets you spell out your decisions about your care ahead of time. Some people create a living will which tells which treatments you want or don't want if you are permanently unconscious or dying. You might include instructions on organ donation, the use of breathing machines, tube feeding, or whether or not you want to be resuscitated.

- **Find local support services.** Look into local services that might be able to provide transportation, nursing care, or even food service to your loved one.
- **Communicate daily.** Call, write, or even Skype every day so that you can feel as though you are an active part of your loved one's life.

CAREGIVER STRESS

Caring for your loved one can be satisfying. It also involves a lot of stress. A caregiver's stress is especially difficult since, like your loved one's illness, it can be chronic and long-term. Without the right amount of help and support, the stress can leave you susceptible to many physical and emotional problems. You, as a caregiver, need care as well. Managing your own mental health is just as important as managing your loved one's health.

SIGNS AND SYMPTOMS OF STRESS

- Anxiety
- Depression
- Trouble sleeping
- Trouble concentrating
- Overreacting to small annoyances
- Worsening or new health issues
- Avoiding friends and social activities
- Loss of interest in things you love
- Insomnia
- Fatigue that won't go away

SIGNS OF CAREGIVING BURNOUT

- Growing resentment toward your loved one
- Constant feelings of helplessness

- Increased infections
- Inability to see hope for the future
- You receive little to no satisfaction from caregiving
- Feeling neglectful of your own needs
- You feel irritable toward your loved one

When you face the injustice of your loved one's illness, there is frequently a desire to try to rationalize or explain the situation. Sometimes, there just isn't an answer. This can make you feel out of control and helpless. It can even make you feel hopeless.

Focus on the things within your control. Instead of dwelling on things out of your control, focus on your reactions and how you deal with the problems, rather than the problems themselves.

Make an effort to be positive. Being positive won't always come natural to you. You sometimes should tell yourself to be positive and focus on small achievements and goals rather than looking at the big picture, which might feel hopeless.

See the forest. Don't stress too much on the little things. Try to avoid tunnel vision and don't let caregiving completely consume your life. Rely on friends, family members, and support networks to help you cope when you feel overwhelmed.

5 THINGS NOT TO SAY TO SOMEONE WITH A CHRONIC ILLNESS

1. "Well, you're looking good anyway. You can't tell anything is wrong with you."

    Although you think you're giving the person a compliment, you're subliminally telling them that they don't appear sick because of their physical appearance. That can register to the person that perhaps you're suspicious that they are sick at all. Instead, you could tell them that they look good and then ask them how they are really feeling.

2. "How do you feel today? You *seem* a lot better."

   Chronic kidney disease is permanent. There is no cure for it. Although the person might have days where they feel better than others, that feeling is temporary. Telling the person that they "seem better" is pressure on them to keep up the good work, even though they have no control over their body. It's also important to listen to their answer when you ask them a question about their health and not answer for them.

3. "What do you <u>need</u> from me?"

   You might think you're being really direct and opening up communication about the person's needs. Sometimes, if they are experiencing guilt or depression, they might not know what they need. It might be hard for them to vocalize their needs at this point. Rather than leaving it an open-ended question, ask specific questions. Ask, for instance, if they're hungry or if they need anything to eat or something to drink. Or if you can help with specific tasks like driving or cooking.

4. "I know how you feel."

   Empathy and sympathy can really help you connect with the person that you're administering care to. Unfortunately for them, you really don't know how they feel. Even if you've gone through something similar, everyone has their own unique experiences. Instead, listen to what the person is telling you and offer sympathy.

5. "I know a remedy that can cure that…"

   Chronic kidney disease is incurable. There are treatments that can help keep it from progressing quickly and, of course, dialysis and a kidney transplant can help lengthen the person's life if the kidneys begin failing completely. To assume that their condition is curable with a simple home or medical remedy, is demeaning and takes away the severity of the illness itself.

The strain of caregiving can be great, particularly if you feel you don't have any control over what you are doing. The feelings associated with caregiving are normal. If you find yourself full of stress and anxiety, however, then you might find that caregiving takes a great toll on your relationships, physical, and mental health. This can cause burnout, or even a breakdown. At that point, it's impossible to take care of anyone, including your loved one. Do take care of yourself and your needs so that you are also able to live a rewarding and fulfilling life.

OVERALL, IT TAKES TIME

Although having a loved one diagnosed with chronic kidney disease might momentarily take the wind out of your sails, it doesn't mean an end to the quality of life you have or want to maintain for them. In fact, you actually have the chance to achieve significant insight into yourself as you move through and cope with the different facets of the disease.

Of course, having a chronic condition of any kind means that you will face challenges along the way. From time to time you may have setbacks. There will be some times that you are able to cope more effectively with your condition than others. There might be days when you want to throw in the towel.

It's important not to give up while you're on your journey. Learn new ways of gaining compassion and respect for yourself and your "new normal" as you redefine and restructure your life around your illness.

You'll also learn new standards in which to measure your accomplishments and expectations. Although you might face limitations that you didn't have to work around in the past, part of rising above the condition means that you recognize that they are more than simply a body and its symptoms. You are able to realize that life can have purpose and meaning even though a body might impose limitations upon some actions.

Instead of seeing yourself without this chronic kidney disease, try to accept the chronic kidney disease for what it is and live in the moment. Take control over what you can; your attitude and outlook on life.

Like grief, adapting to the life with a chronic illness is a process with stages that aren't always linear. You might arrive at acceptance, only to have a setback and experience depression. You'll continuously be challenged to revisit different emotions and issues. Learning healthy coping strategies can permit you to return to the place where you're dedicated to having the best quality of life.

In the face of adversity, it takes a lot of determination and strength to continue fighting. Congratulate and acknowledge yourself for possessing these qualities. Be gentle with yourself. Forgive yourself when you hit a rough patch. Healthy living has as much to do with the way that you think as it does the physical aspects of your health. When you are able to live your life in a meaningful way, you are creating a personal sense of self-worth for both you and the person you are caring for.

CHRONIC KIDNEY DISEASE OVERVIEW

THE WORKINGS OF THE KIDNEY

Our kidneys are amazing multitasking powerhouses inside our bodies. They combine to be the most perfect natural filtering systems that man could ever hope to emulate, and act as 24-hour regulators in the self-contained and most efficient balancing act that is the human body.

Although we are usually given two kidneys, some people are born with just the one, while others donate a kidney to allow for the survival of a family member or friend. Kidney transplant surgeries have become commonplace nowadays.

Our two bean-shaped kidneys are located on either side of the spine in the abdominal cavity in the middle of our back. In order to make room for the liver, the right kidney sits fractionally lower than the left one. They are fist-sized vital organs, 4 or 5 inches in length, that weigh roughly 0.5% of our body weight each.

In their function as a filtering system, our kidneys extract waste and toxic materials from the blood, balance body fluids, and aid in several other important functions of the body.

They receive an amount of blood from the heart that is uneven to their weight. In fact, all of our blood runs through our kidneys –several times a day. The kidneys use this blood flow in order to perform functions such as:

- Remove wastes while regulating the balance of electrolytes as well as the body's calcium levels
- Regulate the body's fluid balance
- Help regulate the acid/base concentration of our blood and stimulate the production of red blood cells
- Help regulate our blood pressure

It is the renal artery that feeds the kidneys with the continuous blood flow. Then they process the blood and send it out cleaned through the renal vein. They create urine which goes down to the bladder trough funnel-shaped bodies known as ureters. The urine then remains in the bladder until it is excreted.

To perform its function of filtering this volume of blood, each of our kidneys has about a million microscopic filters referred to as nephrons. When some nephrons get obstructed or weakened, other nephrons take over, at least for some time. It is feasible that one could lose the bulk of nephron capacity –or as much as 90% of kidney function- without experiencing any kidney disease symptoms.

However, if the problem persists beyond a certain point, it causes a chain reaction of blockages to other nephrons. The result is that the remaining nephrons are overwhelmed, and the individual exhibits symptoms and falls sick.

The method commonly used to measure kidney function and determine the person's stage of kidney disease is known as Glomerular Filtration Rate (GFR) whereby a physician first orders a blood test to measure the serum creatinine level, creatinine being a waste product that emanates from muscle activity. The kidneys normally remove creatinine from the blood, so that if left-over creatinine shows up in undesirable levels, it tells the physician that kidney function is weak.

In order to then come up with a GFR level, a math formula is applied that factors in the person's gender, age, race and their serum creatinine.

In addition, more than half of the patients entering dialysis in the US are deemed malnourished, as reflected in their index of protein nutrition, also known as serum albumin level. This has become a regular measure for kidney disease as well.

Because of the exposure to toxins and other blockages, the kidneys are vulnerable to complications, including infection, blood-clotting disorders, autoimmune kidney disorders, and other problems.

Symptoms and Risk Factors of Kidney Disease

Risk Factors

It has been estimated that diabetes and high blood pressure account for 70% of all individuals with kidney disease. Because sustained high blood sugars over several years can impair blood flow to the kidneys, causing blockages, type 2 diabetes leads the list of risk factors which includes:

- Type 2 Diabetes is the number one cause of kidney failure, so controlling blood sugars and minimizing complications is important to slow down the damage to your kidneys

- High blood pressure is next in line as a high risk factor for kidney problems. Hypertension can exert pressure on large and small blood vessels, including our microscopic and delicate nephrons.
- Age and genetic predisposition are also significant factors, with persons over 60 showing a marked increase in kidney disease over persons of younger ages. People who have kidney issues running in their family are also typically advised to check regularly for irregularities.
- Hardening of the arteries, known as atherosclerosis, and the accumulation of plaque in the arteries that supply the kidneys causes restriction of the blood supply and progressive damage to the kidneys, a condition known as known as ischemic nephropathy.
- Obesity, cardiovascular disease, anemia, smoking, drug abuse, blockages in the blood vessels in our arms or legs (known as peripheral artery disease), and the side effects of medications are but some of the other causes of kidney disease.

Symptoms of kidney disease

It must be said that symptoms of kidney disease may not show up until we have an 85% or even 90% rate of failure in kidney function. Part of the reason is that rarely does kidney disease produce pain that can be related to it.

Symptoms of kidney disease may include one or more of the following:

- Changed urination patterns: may have difficulty urinating, or more frequent urination, pale or darker-colored urine depending on frequency of urinating, possible blood in the urine
- Extra fluid builds up in the body causing swelling in the body's extremities as well as in the face and ankles.
- Anemia and fatigue set in when kidneys start failing and stop promoting the production of oxygen-carrying red blood cells. With less oxygen, the brain and muscle tire quickly and succumb to fatigue.
- Anemia can also be linked to impaired cognitive and immune function, new onset of cardiovascular disease, shortness of breath, feeling cold all the time and diminished quality of life.
- When kidney function starts to fail, some waste is allowed to remain in the bloodstream (uremia). This can cause itching, vomiting, nausea, loss of

appetite, loss of weight and "ammonia breath", i.e. a metallic taste in the mouth.

PROGRESSION AND PREVALENCE OF DISEASE

Kidney disease has long been one of the leading health problems both nationally and worldwide. People develop it for wide-ranging reasons, at times discovering it suddenly and in its advanced stages, while at other times it is diagnosed early on and develops slowly over time —frequently over several decades.

Many people with mild kidney disease thus feel well and can go about their work and lifestyles almost unaffected, while in others the kidneys get progressively worse and degenerate into damaged "end-stage" organs that can no longer multi-task as efficiently. When this happens, waste and toxins start accumulating in their bodies, and the patients become really ill, and life as they know it begins to change.

The best scientific gage of the decline in kidney function can be accomplished by using the declining glomerular filtration rate (GFR) system. Our physician can derive the degree to which the kidneys are damaged from the results of our creatinine, mixed in with our age, gender and other factors. This identifies five stages of chronic kidney disease (CKD) based on the presence of kidney damage:

- **Stage 1 – (GFR at 90 ml/min or higher).** Treatment aims at slowing down the progression of kidney disease and preventing heart and blood vessel complications.
- **Stage 2 – (GFR of 60-89 ml/min).** Kidney function begins its decline, and the stage 1 treatments are to be maintained. Most people are not aware of kidney failure at stage 1 & 2.
- **Stage 3A (GFR of 45–59 ml/min).** Anemia may develop, as well as high blood pressure and fluid build-up. People begin to see a nephrologist on a regular basis to slow down the progress of the disease.
- **Stage 3B (GFR rate of 30–44 ml/min).** Complications continue to set in. People may experience fatigue, sleep problems, and other issues.
- **Stage 4 – (GFR of 15 – 30 ml/min).** Patient develops significant symptoms of kidney disease and approaching kidney failure. You need to prepare for the available options for survival. E.g. for hemodialysis, and need to have your veins readied for regular needle insertions. Alternatively, you will need to have a catheter placed in your abdomen for peritoneal

dialysis. You may also ask close relatives or friends to donate a kidney for a transplant procedure.

- **Stage 5 – (GFR below 15 ml/min).** The kidneys cannot sustain life anymore, and you will need dialysis or transplantation.

Here are some facts and figures on the incidence of kidney disease in the US, courtesy of National Kidney and Urologic Diseases Information Clearinghouse (NKUDIC):

- The incidence of kidney disease is increasing at a more rapid rate in individuals age 60 and over
- The probability of persons who do not have chronic kidney problems being alive 12 months after a heart attack is greater than for those with CKD stage 3 and higher
- By the beginning of 2010, approximately 400,000 End Stage Renal Disease (ESRD) patients were undergoing some type of dialysis and 175,000 ESRD patients were living with a transplanted kidney
- The number of ESRD patients who receive hemodialysis (HD) at a medical center is 10 times greater than the combined number of patients who receive that treatment at home and those who receive peritoneal dialysis
- Transplant patients have a survival rate twice that of dialysis patients
- The total national expenditure for the medical care of ESRD came to $40 billion in 2009
- It costs 3 times as much to treat a patient on hemodialysis than a person with a transplant

Chronic Disease

There are numerous types of chronic illnesses, from Chronic Obstructive Pulmonary Disease (COPD) to diabetes, bronchitis, arthritis and several other conditions. As a result, many affected persons have to endure overwhelming emotional and mental hardships, not to mention the pain and suffering that frequently accompanies their illness. This is happening despite the fact that medicine keeps making significant leaps forward in developing cures as well as pharmaceutical drugs that mitigate the harshest of symptoms.

When the condition is degenerative and irreversible, such as Chronic Kidney Disease (CKD), one of the biggest fears is living with their system's gradual decline, not knowing what the next day will bring.

Patients can be forced to make stressful lifestyle changes that are entirely forced upon them. They have to keep adjusting, month after month -at times week after week when the disease has progressed- to new demands on the little that they are still able to do. In addition, the cost of treatments and medications are also constantly on their minds, depleting their resources, frequently to the bitter end. They run out of everything in their lives -emotions, energy, hope- and they just keep pushing along in desperation.

Chronic Kidney Disease (CKD)

Chronic Kidney Disease (CKD) is a debilitating condition that denotes the gradual, progressive loss of kidney function over time. CKD can end in permanent kidney failure, leaving patients with difficult options, as well as the possibility of death. As the 9th leading cause of death in the US, it is estimated that over 25 million Americans have CKD in varying degrees.

As kidney failure advances and the organ's function is compromised as dangerous levels of waste and fluid accumulate in the body.

Treatments are mostly aimed at slowing down the progression of the disease, and they consist for the most part to treat the underlying causes. The root causes of CKD are diabetes and hypertension in the first place, but also obesity, cardiovascular disease, and other less prevalent risk factors.

CKD is also known as chronic kidney failure, chronic renal disease, or chronic renal failure. It is a health condition that leads to difficult outcomes:

- A distressed quality of life
- Anemia, with multiple consequences
- Possible End-stage renal disease (ESRD)
- Possible heart disease
- Premature mortality

In order to survive, when CKD ends in ESRD, patients may need dialysis (artificial filtering of the blood) or a kidney transplant. Hundreds of thousands of CKD patients undergo dialysis or await a transplant each year.

The early symptoms of CKD can be elusive and almost undetectable. One of the ensuing problems is that it frequently goes unnoticed for years on end. This is something referred to as "the silent period", and it can stretch out to two or more decades. The other problem is that its symptoms can resemble those of the underlying causes, allowing the degeneration in kidney function to progress even further. Many sufferers don't have their CKD diagnosed until kidney failure is fast approaching.

It takes targeted blood and urine tests to confirm the disease, and without such tests, the disease can thus take a long period of time before attaining total loss of function. In fact, most people with CKD never see their disease degenerate to the point of failure.

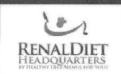

MRS. MURRAY'S STORY

A Story About One Patient's Family and How They Managed With Her Kidney Failure

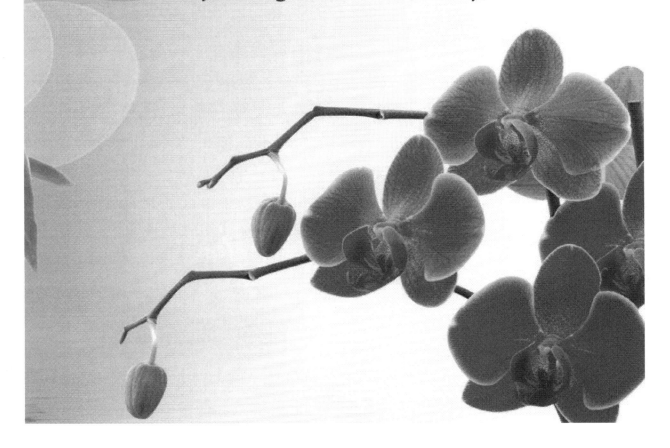

Foreword

Dear Reader,

This book is about Mrs. Murray's caregivers. Mrs. Murray is a gentle and loving woman in her sixties who is suffering from a debilitating chronic illness of the kidneys. Her story really begins in chapter two. But we chose to first tell you everything about her disease, known as chronic kidney disease (CKD).

For the remainder of the book, Sarah, Mrs. Murray's daughter will be talking to you. She is the "primary responsible party" for her mother, meaning that she directs all aspects of her mother's care, including daily caregiving and companionship, doctors, lab tests, medications, home care agency, vendors and whatever else is needed.

You will see how much Sarah, and her distant brother Ben, love their mother. Raised in a home where affection and respect abounded, when their mother becomes ill, they are there, mind, body and soul.

Sarah has a family of her own, including a husband and two teenage boys. She also has a full-time job and has to maintain this balancing act between her job, family and caring for her mother. You will get an insider's peek at how she manages and the system she has in place so as not to get exhausted or overwhelmed. In reality, Sarah represents all daughters, and her brother all siblings who, after being looked after by parents, see the tables turned and now care for their parents.

You will witness Sarah's family's juggling of the different facets of life and how caregiving is achieved. Respite care for the caregivers playing a critical role.

You will read about caregiving, not only from a daughter's point of view, but also from the point of view of a home care agency and a hired caregiver, who is a Certified Nursing Assistant (CNA).

Geoff, a nurse who represents the home care agency, will explain about Mrs. Murray's care from the vantage point of an agency that puts in place caregiving arrangements for dozens of families. How caregiving is done and how much it costs will be discussed, comparing home care to assisted living facilities and nursing homes. Geoff has seen many families of every conceivable type, including Mrs. Murray's type which is governed by genuine tenderness and overriding love.

Janice is Mrs. Murray's live-in caregiver. She works for Geoff's agency and is also highly devoted to Mrs. Murray. She works closely with Sarah and manages Mrs. Murray's day-to-day life, including preparing her meals, taking her out on walks, making sure she takes her medications and providing her personal care tasks, such as grooming, bathing and others.

The symptom of Mrs. Murray's kidney problems that pressures her caregivers the most is her depression. With depression, the world becomes smaller and claustrophobic, and the caregivers are stressed beyond the norm. They constantly need a whiff of fresh air, which brings into play a facet of caregiving that frequently seems like a life-saver. Thus, enters Ben, Mrs. Murray's devoted son and principal respite provider. Respite is when someone relieves a caregiver from her everyday responsibilities, thus enabling the caregiver to take a break and get recharged.

Ben lives out-of-town, but he still plays a pivotal role. He calls his mom regularly and has long, chit-chatty talks with her. She loves those conversations and waits for them passionately. Ben also attends regular teleconferences between all the parties. With Ben being at a certain distance from the day-to-day, his judgment is highly valued. Most significantly however, Ben comes and stays with Mrs. Murray twice a year, for at least 10 or 15 days each time. This allows both caregivers, Sarah and Janice, to take what in caregiving jargon is known as "respite vacations", distinguishing it from "respite breaks" which are for shorter durations. Ben also handles his mother's financial affairs.

You will follow Mrs. Murray's condition as it gradually worsens, causing the family to stare into difficult options.

Those are the characters, and you will live their heroic spirit as well as their many tribulations. They represent formidable tributes to caregivers all over.

Mrs. Murray's Caregivers

Caregivers and caregiving costs

Geoff, Nurse Coordinator

My name is Geoff. I am a Nurse Coordinator at the home care agency hired by Sarah, Mrs. Murray's daughter. When we first started, more than three years ago, none of us had any inkling as to her mother's kidney problems. Sarah simply described her mom as prone to depression and frequently fatigued and without appetite.

Together with Sarah, we decided that 4 hours a day, 5 days a week would do nicely. We would assign a "companion" who would do her light housekeeping, some cooking, laundry and such, and they might also be able to escort her out on errands and perhaps to restaurants or the park.

Companions are the starting aides in a home care agency's arsenal. They are not allowed to undertake any caregiving chores which involves the companion helping the care recipient by using their hands. They can help their patients with chores around the house, outdoor errands, and in providing companionship, or just being there, and doing joint activities, such playing card games, doing puzzles, or reading from books.

When hands-on care is warranted, because the patient needs help with grooming, bathing, incontinence and such, the agency will assign a Certified Nursing Assistant (CNA). This is someone who took the trouble of going to a nursing school or academy, and participating in usually a 120-hour course, at a cost of around $1500, frequently followed by a 50-hour "hands-on" experience at a nursing home. CNAs are the main bastions that home care agencies depend upon to assist seniors (families hiring caregivers privately do not have to abide by these rules).

When we first started, Mrs. Murray didn't need more than that- a few hours a day. At the time, we assigned someone who lasted only a few months, not because she wasn't suitable, but because Sarah thought that her mom now needed 8 hours a day, and our first companion couldn't do the expanded schedule. Turnover in caregiving staff is a real problem.

The cost of a caregiver hired through an agency is not much lower than $20 an hour. Thus for an 8-hour day, it can be $160/day, and assuming the service is needed every day of the year, $160 x 365 days comes to an annual cost of $58,400, to which one naturally has to add the cost of maintaining a home, food, and other expenditures, particularly health costs.

Even if a family hires privately, i.e. not through an agency, the cost is still likely to be upwards of $30,000 a year —exorbitant for most people. And when patients need coverage at night as well, the cost can be that much higher.

This, by the way, compares with the national average daily rate for a private room in a nursing home of roughly $275/day, or a little over $100,000 a year. As for an average Assisted Living Facility (ALF) the cost would be over $55,000/year.

Thus, the seniors who nowadays number over 110 million in the U.S. —and estimated to go up to 120 million by 2020- are for the most part being looked after by their middle-aged children, grandchildren, neighbors, friends and professional nursing assistants, for a total pool of caregivers currently numbering at around 55 million. In most parts of America, help is readily available, though at a high cost.

People refer to this as the "sandwich generation", whereby people in their forties and fifties, typically at or near the peak of their careers, have dual real-time responsibilities to parents as well as children. Even when they can afford to hire part-time or full-time caregivers, they remain their parents' long-term and responsible caregivers. The nation thinks of them as heroes at a time when they think of themselves, at best, as unsung heroes.

Caring for my mother with CKD

Mrs. Murray's daughter, Sarah

My mom means the world to my brother and me. She gave us more love and attention than anyone could hope for from a parent. And she always provided the zest and enthusiasm around the house. Everyone adores my mom: my brother and I, her grandchildren, neighbors who had been close to the family for many years and an array of other relatives and friends.

When mom was widowed some five years ago, she decided, and we all agreed, that she wanted to remain at home for the long run. In time, we sold the old family house and downsized her to a one-floor home in a nice neighborhood. What that did was practically rob her of the friendship of the many neighbors she had cultivated over what seemed to be a lifetime. Sure, one or two still visit her occasionally, but everyone's time seems to be precious. At this time, she has sufficient funds not to have to worry about being able to stay at home over the long run, but we have to think about plan B for the long run.

My mom is sicklier these days than I've ever seen her. Her chronic kidney disease reached stage 3A about a year ago, and although she's been taking her medications without fail, she seems to have declined over the last 12 months. In the last test some 4 weeks ago, her GFR has gone down to 40, indicating CKD stage 3B, and her blood sugars measured over 200 every morning —way too high. Her blood pressure is rarely any better than 160 or 170 over 90. Lately, she has vomited a few times for the first time during her sickness. She complains of nausea and has little or no appetite at times.

The godsend in all this is Janice, mom's caregiver. I don't know what we would do without Janice -and without Geoff as well. At one point Geoff determined to do something about mom's isolation. He and I discussed ways to get her to socialize with people who could become new friends. We tossed around the idea of seeing if mom would be happier in an Assisted Living Facility. She just listened to us and pretended to show interest when I knew she had no interest in such a major undertaking.

Geoff and I thought we could give her a little nudge, and we arranged for her to spend an experimental one week at a nice facility not far from where I live. She lasted three days, and even in those three days, I don't think she struck a conversation with anyone. She had always been reserved, and her health issues made her feel that she would only be "imposing" on someone if she sought their attention. At any rate, that was the end of the facility experiment.

Janice lives-in with mom. She is a Certified Nursing Assistant working for Geoff's agency. She is the best thing that ever happened to our family lately.

I live some 40 miles away from mom, so that a visit to her home takes the better part of a morning or an afternoon. Ben, my brother, calls her two or three times a week, and I spend some time with her usually once during the week, and another time in the weekend. I have two teenage boys and a husband, and I am a full-time

—thus far- teacher at my local high school. I say "thus far" because I can see the day coming when I will have to leave my job to care for mom.

I am usually rushing around non-stop between all my responsibilities, and although everyone says they want to help, I'm still running around all day long every day. And I understand caregivers usually end up suffering from stress and self-neglect, but I always say that to Janice, never thinking of my own predicament.

The professional caregiver

Janice, the hired caregiver

I was introduced to Mrs. Murray about two years ago, when I was still working an 8 hour a day schedule. Later, we had to move to a full-time live-in schedule, which means I stay with her day and night 5 days a week, and Geoff sends another live-in caregiver to fill-in for me during the weekends.

We are of the same age, Mrs. Murray and I, both of us in our mid-sixties. I guess I have become her best friend, apart from her children. She sees how I take care of myself, and this allows her to feel guilt-free when she wants me to care for her.

We moved from a daily, hourly schedule to living-in when she started to have bouts of depression that would last for two or three days on end. Sarah talked her into meeting me from the agency, and that is how I came to work with her.

At first, she did her best to hide her moodiness from me. Sarah noticed that she had begun to let herself go. For example, she wouldn't bother to clean her nails, and I would find her with disheveled hair at times, or wearing her night gown when I showed up in the mid-morning. The first thing I did was instill a schedule in which everything had to be done, daily or weekly.

Every time she brought up the subject of her kidney disease, she mentioned, almost as an aside, that it was an irreversible condition —and that it had no cure. For some reason, she volunteered "irreversible" and "no cure", but never "chronic". I took it as a cry for help, and I heard "chronic" for the first time from her daughter who spelled it out for me. Mrs. Murray had stage 3 Chronic Kidney Disease, or CKD. I had looked after patients with Alzheimer's and all kinds of other maladies, but never CKD, so I asked Geoff to send me reading material on kidney disease. I quickly learned that stage 3 is serious, and in stage 4 doctors start thinking of remedies more drastic than medications.

Presently, she has declined even further. Her blood sugar is always high, as is her hypertension, despite some healthy routines that we follow every day. I cook for her from diabetic cookbooks, and we go outdoors and walk for as long as I can get her to walk without causing strain. My biggest daily issue with her is her moodiness, and the fatigue that has begun to set in. On some days, I have a really hard time encouraging her to get out of bed.

Here are other steps that I have taken to help us:

- Every time we feel stressed, we have a relaxation session of a few minutes. We shut our eyes, and take a few deep breaths, exhaling with deliberation. I call out areas of our bodies that are normally stressed, and we both mentally make the tension unravel.
- We do visualizations, both of us choosing imagery from our respective childhoods. We thus retrograde into adolescence, then puberty, then childhood, and we concentrate on imagery of kids running around, laughing, and screaming with joy. There are times when this visualization puts pleasant smiles on our faces.
- We watch TV together, and sometimes I hold her hand and feel the calmness creep back into her.
- I go out of my way to encourage neighbors and anyone else that Mrs. Murray likes to come and visit, or even to talk on the phone. Her son, Ben, is the best, for when he calls, they talk for a good 20 minutes. And naturally, we wait patiently for the day Sarah visits, making it a special day. Mrs. Murray helps me to create a menu that is appropriate for everyone, and she stays close by while I cook.
- For her depression, I try to take her to the part of the park where there is a pond and we can feed the geese, or we go by car to catch a movie, although sitting for that length of time has become too demanding on her.

At first I didn't want to live-in with a patient. I have my own family, and although I am divorced and my children are more or less on their own, still, I have a home, and it's a sacrifice for me not to be at home after a day's work. This all changed when I started doing the caregiving for Mrs. Murray. She is truly an affectionate, nice person and, what touched me, she is a vulnerable person as well.

Mrs. Murray's Condition Worsens

How it started and where it is now

Mrs. Murray's daughter, Sarah

Mother had never shown any signs or symptoms of kidney disease, or if she had, we would have probably ascribed those to other factors that had nothing to do with her kidneys.

She endured back pain for several years for which she eventually had spinal surgery some six or seven years ago. That was when her creatinine came up at 5.0 and her CKD was first diagnosed. If it hadn't been for her surgery, we would have still been today associating some of the signs we could see, such as swelling in her legs, as well as several other symptoms, to the wrong factors. The only symptoms that we had always tended to with her doctors were her diabetes and hypertension which, we learned, were risk factors for kidney disease and not symptoms of it.

Oddly, if one is going to have CKD at all, it's lucky to have it discovered early on, although mom was already in her late fifties by then. It probably gave her nephrologist the ability to slow down the rate at which her kidneys were degenerating.

I subsequently learned what a nephrologist is and the difference with a urologist. Briefly, a nephrologist, also referred to as "kidney doctor", is a physician who specializes in the diagnosis and non-surgical treatment of kidney disease, including causes of kidney disease, such as kidney stones, hypertension, electrolyte imbalances, and several other risk factors. By contrast, an urologist is a surgical specialist who corrects structural disorders of the kidneys and urinary track with surgery.

It is thought that people in their early 40's lose about 1% of kidney function every year, but with mom, it's been much more rapid than that. At the time of her surgery, I remember that her eGFR (estimated glomerular filtration rate) was at 49, abruptly low. We were told however that they would want to check her GFR to see if it stays that low for a few months —which it did. Today it is in the thirties. The interesting part is that no one in our family had kidney problems before this.

We had thus gone in for spinal surgery and come out with kidney disease – progressive, degenerative and chronic, as we quickly found out, to our utter dismay. My brother Ben lets me handle doctors and tests, and what I never wanted to share with him is that CKD often progresses to stage 5 even when it is diagnosed early on and with aggressive treatment. Stage 5 means her kidneys can no longer sustain life, and she has recourse only to dialysis or transplantation surgery, both stressful options.

I have subconsciously deferred the day when I have to start considering the ramifications of stage 4 and stage 5.

Anyway, since then I made sure mom is well nourished, with particular attention to her glucose and to the protein waste build-up in the blood. I made other lifestyle adaptations that I will let Janice, her angel of a caregiver, describe. Mom sees her nephrologist regularly every three months, taking urine and blood tests to keep an eye on this disease of hers. Her doctor also uses the tests to better calibrate her diet and medications.

We are doing what we can, Ben and I. Ben lives out-of-state and manages all of mother's expenditures and finances. He is an amazing source of support to us. He calls in regularly and makes sure mom is reminded of his love all the time. He also comes and spends two or three weeks with mom at least twice a year, when his work allows it. When he does that, he brings with him an uplifting whiff of fresh air, helping us all. It also enables us to give some respite to Janice. I would like to let Geoff, Janice's Nurse Coordinator, explain how we've managed the respite care schedule we provide to Janice, and its significance.

Lifestyle adaptations for someone with CKD

Janice, the caregiver

I am taken aback by Mrs. Murray's fast deteriorating condition, despite all that we do to keep her healthy. Her blood sugar is relentlessly high, as is her hypertension. At this rate, soon her GFR will go below 30 and her CKD into stage 4. Heaven only knows how high her diabetes and blood pressure would have been without the medications she takes, or the healthy routines that I encourage her to maintain on a daily basis.

Her feet and ankles swell, a condition known as edema, and her skin is always dry and her urine dark. I know that the disease makes bones weak and susceptible to breakages, so I am extra careful where to take her for walks and to make sure the house is safe against falls.

I pick up all clutter, as well as extension cords and long phone lines that go across rooms and have had grab bars installed by the shower, tub and toilet. I have also replaced all bathroom floor mats with slip-free ones and no longer have throw rugs of the type that curl up and cause tripping. At night, I ensure we have night lights in the corridors and areas where she might venture.

I am also told that many of her other symptoms are the result of anemia, which is when an insufficient volume of oxygen is being taken to parts of the body, including the kidneys. This happens when the body is not manufacturing an appropriate volume of hemoglobin or red blood cells, which in turn distribute the oxygen throughout the body.

You can tell that oxygen is lacking sometimes from the pale color it gives the patient. Mrs. Murray has no energy at all and carries on in a lethargic manner. I have to really entice her to even get dressed or prepare for a bath. I guess they call that fatigue. I call it exhaustion.

When I encourage her go for a little walk with me, she is quickly short of breath, and I can tell that she is having a rapid heartbeat.

She recently wakes up with a headache and some dizziness, though not every day. Her doctor tells Sarah that when it comes to diminishing a patient's quality of life, anemia takes the prize.

Anemia stems from insufficient levels of iron and certain vitamins in the body. Thus, whenever we have a teleconference between Sarah, Geoff (my Nurse Coordinator), Ben and I, one of the items we always go over is the medications and dietary plan that Mrs. Murray's doctor prescribed for her and update what I am giving her.

For the production of iron, meat is more easily absorbed into the body than vegetables and fruit, which are good for her diabetes. I watch her overall protein intake, and try to give her high quality meats like beef or liver twice a week, with chicken, pork or shellfish on other days. She does not have a potassium restriction, and spinach and other dark green leafy vegetables are good for all her conditions, so we have those on a daily basis. She likes peas and beans of all types, so I make mixed soups using those, and I buy iron-fortified breads and cereals.

As a caregiver, I can deal with anything, but the thing that I find the hardest to deal with is depression. I am told that many people with CKD also find themselves with bad depressions, probably —one of the reasons I've heard- because of the multiple disorders faced by the patient in their diabetes, hypertension, CKD and possible other disorders.

When I moved in and started living in with Mrs. Murray, she used to have bouts of depression, sometimes lasting for a few days. Now it seems that she is always depressed, and I am constantly hard-pressed to think of ways to relieve her of the bad thoughts inside her mind.

We go out to restaurants and on other projects whenever she feels up to it, which is no more than once every week or 10 days nowadays. I also make sure that she stays in active touch with the support group that her children and I have created for her: friends, Sarah's teenage boys, ex-neighbors, even a real estate agent who helped Sarah and Mrs. Murray find homes in the past.

I am also afraid that she might one day take her own life. I know from my experience with other patients that the short cut to suicide is depression. I therefore stay alert for any such signs which, thankfully, she has not shown yet.

Naturally, her depression is an added pressure on me that I could do without. I have an upbeat personality, however, and lead as healthy a life as I can muster. I eat from what I prepare for her, which is as nutritious as can be, and I take half hour brisk walks at least every day, and frequently mornings and afternoons. Finally, I have an agreement with Sarah and Geoff whereby they promptly arrange for someone to fill-in for me whenever I feel stressed. Respite care is important.

Caring for a caregiver

Geoff, Nurse Coordinator

People don't realize, but in my job as a nurse supervisor, when I go on client visits in homes where we look after someone, I am equally interested in checking on the patient's wellbeing as well as that of our caregiver.

With Mrs. Murray, mine is typically a routine visit in which I take her vital signs and chat with her for a little while to try to pick up on possible signs of anything that raises a flag.

My task is different with Janice, and particularly with a caregiver looking after a patient with dementia or, as with Mrs. Murray, a patient with depression. Note that I haven't mentioned the CKD, for that is relatively straightforward for me to deal with as a nurse, checking vital signs, medications and diets, updating the patient's chart, and discussing the patient's condition with the caregiver.

It is Mrs. Murray's depression that concerns me, for I know how exhausted and overwhelmed a caregiver can get. For their hard work and devotion to their patients, caregivers frequently pay a high toll in terms of emotional and physical stress. They typically can't find the time to look after themselves, and while they can put perfect order in their patients' lives, caregivers frequently can't balance between work and their personal or family needs.

I even worry about Sarah, Mrs. Murray's daughter who, although she is at a distance, cares for her mother to the point where life must be extremely stressful for her as well. I once tried to help her get some respite by placing her mom –even temporarily- in an assisted living facility, but Mrs. Murray didn't like it at all and wanted to get back home quickly.

Assisted living facilities are frequently used in that way, to give respite to family caregivers for a specified period of time. With an ALF, as we refer to them, there are nurses and CNAs to look after residents, so that family caregivers can remove themselves entirely from their caregiving responsibilities and do whatever they have to do to recharge their emotions and energy.

Naturally, it doesn't help much if you burn out first and then take a vacation. Respite breaks are intended to achieve the exact opposite of that. Respite breaks should be part and parcel of caregiving duties from day one. You know that the job is going to wear you out, and you know how easy it is to break down and be overwhelmed, so the smart thing to do for any caregiver is to factor in respite breaks, for the sake of their "sanity" or wellbeing. And a step up from respite breaks are respite vacations.

This is what Ben, Mrs. Murray's son, offers to both Janice as well as his sister by coming twice a year and spending roughly two weeks with his mother. They learn to schedule pleasant things to do for Sarah while he's in town. She takes respite vacations, even when she stays at home. The rules are that no one can call her during these breaks, thus letting her mind wander truly away from it all and into more uplifting activities. Janice also takes time away with her family.

Hiring an agency like ours provides respite peace of mind in the sense that if the caring members of the family were to have to suddenly travel or not be there for a while, the agency takes over completely. In fact, rarely have I had to deal with someone like Sarah who is passionately involved with her mother's affairs on a daily basis.

Mrs. Murray's options

Sarah

I tear up every time my mind dwells on where we're headed. Mom is so delicate, so fragile; she certainly doesn't deserve any of this.

Based on mom's rapid decline into a GFR (glomerular filtration rate) in the low 30's, Ben and I are thinking that mom will reach End Stage Kidney Disease, which is also referred to as End Stage Renal Disease (ESRD), within 12 to 18 months. That will be when her kidneys will stop being able to flush out the waste and fluids, and when diets and medications will no longer do the job.

Doctors frequently like to delay the next steps as long as possible since they carry the risks of complications. But the need for a transplant or dialysis becomes imminent.

My initial thoughts together with my brother are that we go with dialysis, a process that attempts to keep the patient alive and functioning for as long as possible. We would have normally preferred a transplant for which both Ben and I would have been more than willing donors. But mom's condition is too fragile, and we think she wouldn't be able to sustain a major surgery such as a transplant.

We decided to ask her doctor to bring up this subject delicately and lay out the options so that mom can take part in the decision-making process. That visit went well, for every time her doctor stopped, I prodded for more information of the type that mom needs. Then on our next call to Ben, we were able to bring up the subject openly, and although mom kept quiet most of the time, at least she now knows what all of us are facing.

Kidney dialysis has the task of taking over from the now defunct kidneys their function of removing from the body waste substances and fluids.

Although there are two main types of dialysis, Ben and I promptly agreed that hemodialysis (HD) is the pathway we would take. It is also preferred to peritoneal dialysis by a factor of ten to one. The two systems are:

Hemodialysis – This is where blood is pumped out of the patient's body and goes through an artificial kidney known as a dialyzer. One of the problems of this method is that blood has to be pumped out of a main source, so one can either have it pumped out by way of a catheter that is placed in one of the patient's main blood veins or, alternatively, a junction can be created surgically between a vein and an artery in the patient's arm. After filtration in the dialyzer, the blood is returned to the patient.

Peritoneal dialysis – is performed by surgically placing a special, soft, hollow tube into the peritoneal cavity of the abdomen near the navel. This contains a vast network blood vessels, and the patient's blood is filtered there by infusing a dialysis solution into the tube and draining it out repeatedly to remove the unwanted waste and fluids.

In the options that Ben and I reflected upon, we thought about dialysis at home, for they have nowadays home-use dialysis machines that make dialysis at home more practical for some. When the time comes however, we think we prefer for mom to go to a dialysis clinic that would transport her back and forth and look after her for the duration, giving Janice a mini break. We figure that at a clinic she can meet other patients rather than remain cooped up at home. It's also the option that her doctor suggested to me when I recently asked him about it.

Mom would have to undergo hemodialysis three times a week, each session lasting for at least three hours.

We really haven't made iron-clad decisions on this subject as yet. We have been pushing it off for obvious reasons. I will therefore have more to tell you later about dialysis and transplant surgery.

Mrs. Murray's Depression

Letting Janice go

Sarah

I am going through a very unsettling period involving major changes in our lives. I just pray that I stay strong and see us through those changes as calmly as possible.

It is all about mom's finances. She has been spending at a non-sustainable rate over the last few years. Ben tells me that her household expenditures on utilities, food and medications come to about $1,200 a month, whereas what we pay Geoff's agency for Janice and for the other fill-in caregivers comes to a whopping $5,000 a month.

Every time I talk to Geoff I bring out the possibility of hiring privately. He has become a dear friend with whom I can discuss something like that which in theory goes against the best interests of his agency. He has no qualms about it however since we've been great clients for a long time.

It turns out that I can hire a full-time live-in caregiver like Janice for about $100 a day, or $3,000 a month, a good saving over what the agency charges us. He explains to me however that there are several obstacles in the way. For a start, I would have to run recruiting ads, talk to caregivers on the phone, interview the ones who sound reasonably qualified, review all their paperwork, run criminal background checks on them, call their references, and then hope that mom will like the final candidate that I select. If she doesn't, I have to do all that again.

In addition, Geoff cautions me that privately hired caregivers have a high turnover. They have a tendency to leave the job within two or three months of the start. Apparently they get lured by better jobs, perhaps because a job is closer to where the caregiver's home is, or because it's an easier patient to look after. Also, they frequently leave because of the lure of a live-out job that would allow them to go home at night rather than live-in with the patient.

At any rate, any one of those eventualities would leave me in a quandary. Geoff finally cautions me that if I hire privately, I wouldn't have the agency to fall back on with fill-in caregivers. Every time the privately hired caregiver wants a day off, or the weekend, or has an emergency and needs to take off, I would have to drop everything and rush to mom's side.

No wonder, I thought to myself, so many families provide their loved ones with care from within the family. I remember the statistic that claims that there are approximately 50 million family caregivers looking after 110 million aging seniors in the U.S., and both those numbers are on the increase.

Because of the money situation getting tight, and because of the high cost of a hired caregiver, I have decided to leave my job and bring mom to live with my husband, our two boys and I. This plan naturally involves letting Janice go and selling mom's house.

Ben and my husband desperately tried to figure out some other path for us to take. They particularly hate for me to leave my work and become mom's full-time caregiver, a limiting proposition no matter how one looks at it. The prospect of nurses and technicians coming and going at the home of a dialysis patient isn't exactly joyful. In addition, although no one mentions it, I am only too aware that we are all going to lose a good measure of privacy when mom moves in with our family.

The ones who stand to lose a lot in all this, my husband and my boys, are squarely behind me. They keep saying: "If you think it is the best way to go, count us in."

Ben and I talk almost daily, with him exploring the option of selling mom's house and renting a place for her close to where I live, and then perhaps being able to make do with hiring a caregiver privately for only a few hours a day. I just don't see how that can work. If I am in going to be at the mercy of a caregiver we can ill afford, I'm better to take on the caregiving duties myself.

However, all of this is easier said than done. I do not in any way relish the task of telling mom and Janice about any of it. Mom is going to be devastated, as if she doesn't have enough on her plate as things are. She has grown to depend entirely on Janice, and sometimes I discover her telling Janice things she never brings up in my presence, showing me how close they have become. I have no idea how she is going to respond to the changes I have to talk to her about, particularly in view of her depression that keeps worsening almost day by day.

As for Janice, I tear up every time I think about letting her go. She has been a model caregiver and friend for both mom and I, but particularly for mom. She treats mom with a gentle and loving touch that is at times just marvelous to observe. She can find any number of jobs she wants through Geoff's agency or on her own, and I will give her the best possible recommendations for that. However, that's not the point. It is more a matter of how attached Janice is to her patient and suddenly, when mom needs her the most, Janice is being let go.

We have a doctor's appointment for mom next week, at which time they will run tests to check on her CKD. I have a feeling that her GFR will have dropped below 30, i.e. reflecting a deterioration from stage 3B to stage 4. If this proves to be the case, it will put an increased sense of urgency on our plans.

In any case, I decided to talk to mom and Janice right after we get her test results, probably by the end of next week. Ben and I see no point in raising the alarm sooner than that. Also, even if we have to start taking the various steps of putting the house on the market and moving mom to my home, I don't see that happening for another four weeks at least. That will give Janice a chance to transition mom to my care.

Mrs. Murray's depression

Geoff
We established earlier that Mrs. Murray suffers from anemia, a disorder that people sometimes refer to as "tired blood". More accurately though, anemia is when the hemoglobin level is low. There is a deficiency of red blood cells that take oxygen to body tissues and cleanse them of carbon dioxide. Anemia is the most common of blood disorders in the U.S. and a particularly common disorder among the elderly and those with CKD.

We know that Mrs. Murray is anemic, and when her symptoms of fatigue started showing up in a more advanced way, we naturally attributed it to anemia. And yet, there are several other causes of fatigue such as emotional stress, insomnia, physical exhaustion (meaning over-exerting muscles during workouts), the psychological effects of a chronic illness, and a variety of medical problems, not least of which is depression.

With Mrs. Murray, I believe we can promptly rule out physical over-exertion, leaving us with just about every other common risk factors.

It is not difficult to recognize when a patient is fatigued, yet it is frequently a different matter altogether to pinpoint the processes responsible for this condition. Mrs. Murray's fatigue is an overwhelming feeling of tiredness. At times, it is debilitating enough to stop her from doing everyday things like getting out of bed and putting on something to wear.

Fatigue, as experienced by Mrs. Murray, is best described as hitting a brick wall. It is all consuming and relentless, rendering the rest of "life" almost unbearable.

Why does she feel this way? Well, she feels this way because of a combination of sleeplessness, anxiety, a pessimistic outlook to most things in life and, most significantly, depression. Mrs. Murray also harbors a feeling of guilt in view of the distress she believes she causes to those who love and care for her, yet her children love being able to do this.

Depressed patients often report being detached from the world around them, and with a lack of interest in the things they have always liked. Feeling constantly tired is a common, if unhealthy, part of a too-busy life. Feeling listless and apathetic for weeks, months, or years at a time are signs of depression.

A European study showed that depression and fatigue fuel each other in a vicious cycle, with patients experiencing depression being that much more likely to experience fatigue, and patients suffering from fatigue being significantly more vulnerable to experience depression. While the researchers were quick to point out that the two conditions have separate causes, they appear to feed off of each other and often co-exist in the same patient.

Mrs. Murray's depression is at the center of Sarah's and Janice's concerns these days, and it is proving difficult for them not to get pulled down into the sadness she feels. For Ben, it is different. Not only is he at a distance from their daily grind, but Sarah also tells me he always had an upbeat personality that insulated him against troubling news and people's bad moods. He remains calm and thoughtful even through the decision-making process that involves such drastic changes as to where Mrs. Murray is going to live and Janice having to relinquish her caregiving duties.

Sarah and Janice don't unfortunately share in Ben's uplifting disposition. During a recent visit at a time when Sarah also happened to be at her mother's, I found them both in a morose state of mind, the glumness oppressing all around the house.

I discuss Mrs. Murray's depression with Sarah every time we speak on the phone. I am only too familiar with the many manifestations of depression, the disorder increasing in prevalence with the aging population that my agency serves.

In the last decade or so, many mental health specialists have refuted the long-held view that depression results from a deficiency of one neurotransmitter such as serotonin or dopamine. They consider that notion as being both simplistic and inaccurate. This thesis has opened up other possibilities as being causes of depression.

Thus, one of the many things I discuss with Sarah is the relationship between depression and sleep. There is an abundance of research now to show that depression worsens with people who have an insufficient number of hours of sleep per night, and that results are improved for individuals who get 7 to 9 hours' sleep, versus those who manage only six hours or less. This rang a bell since I know from Sarah that Mrs. Murray frequently complains of her insomnia and it's effects.

The symptoms of depression that I am familiar with almost without exception apply to Mrs. Murray: loss of weight (she has been losing weight consistently in the last few months), loss of appetite (the same), loss of cognitive abilities (she has been exhibiting some signs of short term memory loss), thoughts of being unworthy of people's attentions (she is always pent up with feelings of guilt towards those who care for her), and generally being lethargic and showing no interest in wishing to undertake activities that up to now had been favorites.

When these symptoms persist over several weeks and months, the diagnosis becomes one of Major Depressive Disorder. That is when it becomes a major struggle to do things like getting out of bed and going through the motions of getting dressed and looking after personal hygiene and grooming. The day becomes mired in lethargic motion and drudgery.

Of course, with CKD, there is a natural inclination to just blame the chronic disease for the depression. Chronic disease, after all, is a known lead in to depression. Also, depression among patients with CKD may be somewhat inflated because of the presence of co-occurring conditions that result in CKD such as diabetes, hypertension and heart disease.

At one point, I brought to Sarah's attention something that I read in a medical review, something which I subsequently linked in my mind to her hurried plans regarding her mother, Janice, and all the rest of it. This is about people over 60 with CKD who were also diagnosed with major depression and who were in poor health. It was not something pleasant to report, but I felt I had to share this with her.

In Dallas, TX at UT Southwestern Medical Center, researchers found that patients with CKD who have also been diagnosed with major depression are twice as likely to be hospitalized and to progress to long-term dialysis treatments -or die within a year- as those who are not depressed.

"Chronic kidney disease patients with depression have poorer health outcomes than those without depression, even after adjusting for other factors that determine poor outcomes in these patients, such as other medical diseases, anemia and low albumin levels," said Dr. Susan Hedayati, lead author of the study. She went on to alert physicians to screen CKD patients for depression, particularly in view of the fact that depression is in any case associated with poor quality of life.

In previous reports, Dr. Hedayati found that one in five CKD patients is depressed before beginning long-term dialysis therapy, and that for patients already on dialysis who also suffered from depression, the outcomes are that twice as many CKD patients will need to be hospitalized or die within a year than those who don't have depression.

This study also raised the prospect of viewing all antidepressant treatments for patients with kidney disease with caution and not assuming that the efficacy of such treatments is going to be the same as in patients who do not have kidney issues.

Other researchers have come to conclusions similar to those in Dr. Hedayati's study. A 10-year US study of more than 5500 people aged 65 years or older found new onset of end-stage renal disease was more common in patients with depressive symptoms. In addition, individuals with CKD were 20% more likely to experience depression than their counterparts who did not have kidney disease.

With 26 million annual CKD patients in the U.S., and with 40% of them with major depression, that puts more than 10 million Americans at greater risk than others who have CKD but are not depressed. Of those in dialysis treatment, the number of CKD patients who also have major depression has been estimated to be 50%.

Dr. Timothy Mathew, medical director at Kidney Health Australia, said the ongoing research reminds us that depression is more frequent in people with CKD, and that it is associated with rapid worsening of kidney function and accelerated need for dialysis.

Says Dr. Mathew: "It is a reminder that all practitioners involved with care of people with early or moderate CKD should look for and actively manage depression that is easily masked by the other symptoms of reduced GFR – such as tiredness, lack of concentration and irritability,"

Exactly what Mrs. Murray complains from: tiredness, lack of concentration, and some short-term memory loss. When you learn that your kidneys are deficient, and that they will only keep functioning for a little while longer, it is only normal to feel angry, fearful and depressed.

In consultation with me, Janice is putting on a classic case of treatment with lifestyle adaptations for Mrs. Murray's depression. Here is what she does:

- She is relentless with the nutritious food that she prepares, sticking to dietary advice given by Mrs. Murray's doctor.
- When the weather permits, they spend at least 30 minutes every day outside in the fresh air, as much of this time walking about for exercise.
- She surrounds Mrs. Murray with sounds and smells that are pleasant; she lets the sunshine in, and she frequently plays some of Mrs. Murray's favorite music.
- She keeps Mrs. Murray's support group motivated, inviting those who can to come visit, and ensuring that the others call regularly.

- She invites Mrs. Murray to play scrabble, cards and other games of the mind that will make her patient think.

As for treatment for depression, Mrs. Murray's doctors definitely want to stay away from adding new medications to the list she already takes for diabetes and hypertension as this may only add burden to her failing kidneys.

In fact, only a relatively small number of CKD patients with depression are treated with antidepressant medications or psychotherapeutic methods. The reasons for this low treatment rate boil down to a lack of scientific data that support the safety of various treatment regimens in CKD patients. Mrs. Murray has also not been advised to consult with a counselor.

Transplant Surgery and Dialysis

We first examined transplant surgery

Geoff

Sarah asked me if I would go with them to this latest visit to Mrs. Murray's nephrologist, which I was happy to do. Since the results of the blood and urine tests would take a day or two, the discussion revolved entirely around the relative merits of a kidney transplant procedure compared to dialysis treatment.

For transplant surgery, the physician first explained that the patient can receive a kidney from a cadaver, i.e. a deceased person, or from a live person, usually a blood relative or friend whose blood type is compatible with that of the recipient. This is known as a living transplant, and donors can continue living happily with their remaining kidney.

A kidney transplant is commonly desirable for people with end stage renal disease (ESRD), an irreversible permanent condition of kidney failure that often requires surgery or dialysis. This failure may be caused by diabetes or hypertension, repeated urinary infections, toxins and obstructions, and a number of diseases and disorders.

This compatibility issue involves extensive testing that can only be accomplished by a transplant team whose task is to determine eligibility for transplant. The team includes a transplant surgeon, a transplant nephrologist, an anesthesiologist, a transplant nursing staff, a social worker and a mental health therapist. There are times when a dietitian is also part of the team.

I noticed that Mrs. Murray was not paying too much attention, probably because Sarah calmed her down earlier by telling her that she wasn't about to go through a procedure like this. At one point, she also said that she was getting tired, so Sarah took her out and settled her in the front reception area where she wouldn't have to listen to the details of the transplant procedure.

The transplant team will first go through the recipient's information from interviews, medical history, and past as well as current notes from the patient's nephrologist.

They will do the same to the donor (living-related transplant) to ensure that they are in good health and that their blood type is compatible with the recipient's. The donor must also satisfy the team that they are in good enough psychological condition to undertake such a step.

They would then look at the latest blood tests with the aim of establishing whether there is a good donor match. A good match improves the recipient's chances of not rejecting the donor kidney.

Diagnostic tests are typically performed to evaluate the recipient's kidneys as well as their health in general. X-rays, ultrasound procedures, kidney biopsy, and dental examinations are all likely candidates for thorough examination. Women would undergo a Pap test, gynecology evaluation, and a mammogram.

Psychological issues involved in organ transplantation would also be discussed. This is the part that made Ben and Sarah decide they would not consider the transplant route for Mrs. Murray. They are somehow convinced she wouldn't survive the ordeal. Stress, and the recipient's ability to absorb additional stress, is assessed. Apparently, this issue, including the recipient's fortitude of character, can significantly impact the outcome of a transplant.

Once everything has been deemed positive, the donor and recipient can choose their own date for the procedure, as long as the transplant team's schedule can accommodate that date. After that, the only preparation needed if the recipient is on dialysis is to have one more treatment before the operation. Whether on dialysis or not, both donor and recipient are asked to fast for at least 8 hours before the operation.

As with other surgeries, transplant procedures carry risks, primarily to do with infections of the kidneys, bleeding, and blockage of blood vessels to the donor kidney. There are times when all goes well except that the new kidney doesn't function.

Add to that complications that arise from the recipient's immune system that gages the new kidney as an invading object and fights it as it would a virus of infection. Rejection of the donor kidney ensues and to prevent that, immunosuppressant medications are used of the type that can trick the recipient's immune system into accepting the foreign object. The recipient will thereafter be given antirejection medications for life.

This is a significant procedure that requires the recipient to remain in hospital for several days. I ended up siding with Ben and Sarah and am frankly relieved that Mrs. Murray is not going to risk a transplant. She is far too fragile and would not be able to withstand the procedure itself, never mind complications that may arise.

Home Hemodialysis (HHD)

Sarah

Mom's GFR came back at 26, which is CKD stage 4. Her levels of urea and creatinine were at the highest yet, and her nephrologist told me that she is fast heading toward renal failure.

He wants her to have a chest X-ray to rule out pulmonary edema or fluid retention in the lungs, as well as an ultrasound scan to determine if there are any blockages in the urine flow. He also wants me to come back, without mom, so that he can give me the necessary referrals and instructions for the dialysis. I explained that we were about to move mom from her home to mine, to which he simply urged me not to delay.

A decision was subsequently made by Ben, mom and I. We are now intent on going with the nocturnal version of Home Hemodialysis. I will explain why we decided on that option in a minute. First though, a little of what I learned about dialysis, and HHD in particular.

Hemodialysis involves the removal of waste substances and excess fluid from the patient's body with the use of a dialysis machine. When hemodialysis is performed at home it is referred to as Home HD, or HHD. During an HHD treatment, blood is removed from the body and pumped by a machine through a dialyzer. The blood is then filtered through the dialyzer several times and finally returned to the patient's body.

More precisely, the process requires a dialysis machine, a dialyzer, dialysate and some blood lines. The term "dialysate" involves large quantities of very clean water. Usually, a water treatment system is used, and in it the water goes through a series of filters until it reaches a level clean enough for dialysis. At that point, the water is delivered to the dialysis machine where it is mixed with a special concentrate and becomes referred to as dialysate. It takes roughly 1500 liters of water for each treatment.

The dialysis machine is the engine that takes charge of the treatment. It is prepared with lines for blood flow, dialysate and a dialyzer, and the patient, or someone assisting the patient, can program the machine for the number of hours desired as well as the amount of water to be removed. The machine also has safety features that can detect air and blood clots.

The dialyzer, aka the artificial kidney, is an amazing machine that does the cleansing work that is normally left up to the kidneys to do. The machine pumps the blood through the blood lines to the dialyzer and then back to the patient. The filter is roughly 11 to 13 inches long and contains thousands of tiny fibers with microscopic holes through which the blood travels. The blood then travels through these hairs and is cleansed by the surrounding dialysate.

Now some preparatory work is needed on the patient, namely to create what is known as a fistula, i.e. when an artery is connected directly to a vein. This fistula is created in an outpatient procedure by a surgeon, usually 6 weeks or longer ahead of the first dialysis treatment. The blood thus pours out of the artery and enlarges slightly the vein, or the fistula, in which two needles are inserted, the first to remove the blood, and the latter to return it cleansed.

Putting in the needles is usually the most feared part of the effort, although the fear dissipates once patients insert the needles by themselves, or the same person assisting the patient can insert them every time. Needles are sharp and large, but people soon get over this. In our case, I will have to do it for mom, and I really don't see any problem there.

For treatments at home, the patient can lie or sit next to the HD machine if the HD is done during the daytime. The patient can watch TV, read, or participate in whatever is going on in the home. Nocturnal treatments involve a slower and longer treatment while the patient sleeps. It is common for each treatment to last six to eight hours, and it is the patient's doctor who will prescribe the number of times per week, between three and seven.

The added benefit of nocturnal HHD treatments is that they have a mitigating effect on headaches and nausea commonly associated with other treatments because a smaller amount of fluid is removed with each treatment, and the excess fluid is removed at a slower rate and over a longer period than in other types of dialysis that have shorter treatments.

In comparison, so called "in-center" dialysis treatments are more commonly done three times a week and for four to six hours each time.

In our case, we chose the nocturnal type of HHD, letting mom do it at night, hopefully while she rests or sleeps. This is one of the main advantages of home HD in that the time of day and other requirements of each treatment are controlled by patients and their caregivers rather than by rigid appointments at the medical center. By dialyzing longer, as is common in the nocturnal HHD, dietary restrictions the patient was on previously are relaxed.

Dialysis has become common place and different people use it in different manners. For example, some may undergo 5 or 6 shorter treatments a week if they have a schedule to sustain in another aspect of their lives, such as a job or recreational activity.

Prompted by mom's nephrologist who gave me some reading material specially addressed to the families of dialysis patients, I started reading up on HHD which began in the early 1960's in cities on both sides of the "pond" (Atlantic Ocean) and has since undergone numerous refinements and improvements, as well as a vast lowering of costs.

Nocturnal HHD requires permanent vascular access, typically in the arm, and it does not offer the patient the opportunity to socialize with other patients at the center, or to be assisted by nurses or doctors. However, this type of treatment has health and lifestyle benefits that include:

- Has less limitations on diet and fluid intake
- Requires less medications for hypertension and for lowering phosphates
- Allows travel with portable equipment
- Encourages patients to be involved in own care
- Can regularly have free daytimes

Like HHD, Peritoneal dialysis (PD) need not involve the patient having to go to the dialysis center. Patients can be assisted, or they can help themselves, at home or wherever else they may be. However, this form of dialysis must be performed on a daily basis.

PD first came about in the 1980's, and it works by using the patient's "peritoneum", which is a membrane that lines the walls of the abdominal cavity. A cleansing liquid, known as the dialysis solution, is then inserted into the abdomen through a tube known as a catheter. The peritoneum allows wastes and excess fluid to pass from the blood into the abdomen and the dialysis solution. The dialysis solution is then drained, several times per treatment and the wastes and fluids are discarded appropriately.

Usually, the draining maneuver takes a good half hour. During the actual PD, the dialysis solution is kept inside the abdomen for 5 or 6 hours.

I Have Become Mom's Caregiver

The Caregiver's Predicament

Janice

What happens to a professional caregiver when her patient transitions to some kind of living facility?

With Mrs. Murray being taken tomorrow to an assisted living facility (ALF), this issue that is frequently discussed between friendly Certified Nursing Assistants (CNAs) came to my mind. Sarah and Ben decided, and their mother concurred, that she would be better off in an ALF for three or four weeks while the movers take her personal belongings to Sarah's and while Mrs. Murray's house is "staged", i.e. painted and prepared for showing to prospective buyers.

At any rate, I will be bidding the family farewell tomorrow morning, after nearly four years.

So, I told Geoff that I would like to take a couple of weeks off and then start a new job.

My heart is dismayed at leaving Mrs. Murray. I cared for her like a good friend. I have accustomed Mrs. Murray to talking. She is naturally withdrawn, but if one gives her the time and listens attentively, she will talk. She will get things off her chest and feel better afterwards. We do that for hours at times, and I am just wondering who is going to listen to her in the future.

I will have to acclimatize to life without Mrs. Murray. Perhaps my new job will permit me to visit her occasionally.

Sarah

I made an appointment with mom's surgeon for him to prepare the fistula on mom's arm for dialysis. A fistula is the surgically crafted junction between a vein and an artery. Since this needs to be done several weeks prior to the first dialysis treatment, I wanted to get it done ASAP, as no one can tell when mom will reach end stage renal failure. We better be ready for when that happens.

After the outpatient procedure, I am taking mom to spend some time at an assisted living facility where she stayed once for a few days. This was Ben's idea, and now that everything seems imminent, I really thank him for it. I could never have coped with everything that is happening simultaneously.

I have movers bringing some of mom's belongings to my home. I have to get her house painted and "staged" for prospective buyers and then put it on the market. I also have to get her room ready at home, where I need to set up the dialysis machine and other equipment. And finally, I have to get mom and myself knowledgeable and ready in the smooth performance of a dialysis treatment. This last task scares me the worst, for I have visions of messing up and seeing mom suffer in my incompetent hands.

I also have to ensure that mom is reasonably happy at the assisted living, where I will have to visit on a daily basis. I wish we could have somehow kept Janice for a few more weeks, but that simply wasn't practical. I asked mom what gift we should get for Janice, and all she could do was begin to cry. With Geoff's help, I ended up buying Janice a beautiful winter coat and will give her $500 in cash when I say goodbye to her in the morning.

Geoff

Moving from a chronic disease to dialysis is frequently not such a scary step, for living with a chronic disease is itself just as worrisome. In the past I've had a couple of clients on dialysis, and if my memory serves me, they adjusted and coped fairly well after only a few weeks. Naturally, with Mrs. Murray being as predisposed to depression and fatigue as she is, this might give her an excuse to let go and simply not make the effort to adjust.

In that regard, she would probably have fared better going to a dialysis center where she would meet friendly nursing staff and many of the other patients repeatedly to the point where she might have felt good about it and made some friends. All it takes to perk up sometimes is to look into other patients' eyes and see that they are comfortable with their treatments and reasonably content. I can see where the plan that Ben and Sarah made for their mom made financial and practical sense, but doing the treatments at a center would give Mrs. Murray a chance to come out of her saddened shell. Instead, she is now going to be cooped up at home somewhat.

I am also afraid for her because, like most people, she probably knew nothing about dialysis until Sarah and Ben started talking about it. Also, she was there when the doctor explained in great detail what it would imply, how things work, and what patients experience emotionally at first. If only Mrs. Murray can accept that dialysis will improve her quality of life.

Tomorrow, the surgeon will need to make an access into Mrs. Murray's blood vessels. I am thinking that it is quite possible that Mrs. Murray blood vessels may not be up to the task, in which case the surgeon may do a graft, i.e. use a plastic tube to join a vein and an artery under the skin.

The amount of waste she has in her body, her weight, and the amount of fluid gained in between sessions will determine the length of her HHD treatment.

On the plus side, nocturnal treatments will offer Mrs. Murray the chance to sleep for several hours while the treatment is underway, thereby avoiding the possibility of being bored during the long hours of dialysis during the daytime. People who go to dialysis clinics pass the time chatting or watching TV or reading.

At first, Mrs. Murray is likely to be overcome with fear and dialysis-related stress. These are common feelings shared by many when they first go on dialysis. Everything about dialysis is new and therefore scary; particularly the big needles and watching one's blood go through the dialyzer. As the treatments roll by however, people get over these initial fears and in time get comfortable with the process. I hope Mrs. Murray quickly makes such adjustments. It will impact her drastically, but the treatments will keep her alive.

The reason I'm being guarded about Mrs. Murray's outcome has to do with what I read about the mental health condition of people on dialysis: apparently over half of them are afflicted with depressive episodes. That doesn't bode well at all.

There is a "before" and a "since" notion about dialysis, new norms that one has to accept and believe in. As to one's physical health, patients with ongoing treatments have to maintain a healthy lifestyle as before, and better. In Mrs. Murray's case, her diabetes needs to be attended to, and although the treatments will mitigate her hypertension to a small degree, she will still need to take medications just like in the past.

Individuals on dialysis are encouraged to remember that none of their prior conditions will go away as a result of the treatments, and that they need to lead a healthy life and to talk to their dietitian about creating a nutritious diet whereby they can have the right daily amount of protein, fluids, calories, vitamins and minerals, a diet that is adjusted for their particular needs. Add to that plenty of physical activity and 7 to 9 hours of sleep if possible.

The best natural remedy for depression is to stay close to the people whose company you cherish, and socialize, talk an laugh as much as possible with them. Laughter is the most perfect natural antidote to depression and worth every effort.

Parting words

Mrs. Murray's son, Ben
I guess we have entered the period where our lives have been tossed up in the air, subject to settling back down in new ways. I will be flying in to be with my family next week and will be able to spend at least two or three weeks helping Sarah and holding mom's hand.

I called Janice and made sure to be able to see her, even after mom went to the ALF. I am especially grateful for the way that she sustained mom all those years. We would come and go, but Janice was the constant in mom's lfie.

I thought the idea of the ALF for mom for a few weeks to give everyone, particularly Sarah some breathing room. It is not easy to have so much happening and be preparing at the same time to use needles on mom and to operate the dialysis system on her own at home. I wanted to be there when she and mom received the necessary training which I gather is extensive.

The sale of the house will help considerably. I gathered from talking to the real estate agent that this is typical of a home that was purchased many years ago for under $20,000 that will now fetch more than 10 times as much. She was telling me that many of the families she helps use the proceeds from the house towards the upkeep of aging parents who outlived their savings. Older seniors who planned for life up to the early eighties are now living well over that, causing difficulties for their children who also have young ones going through college.

I hope mom does well at the ALF. I need her to be in a positive frame of mind in this coming period. The treatments will give her enough cause for being depressed without adding her natural down disposition to it. And I hope that the new blood pressure medicine given her by her doctor does the job. Hypertension and kidney disease are mutually affecting, as is diabetes, so I will want to make sure she is taking care of herself during my visit. She should maintain blood pressure at no more than 140 over 90 prior to the treatments, and further down slightly during treatments.

Also, mom, as far back as I can remember, suffered from diabetes, which is the biggest single risk factor for kidney disease. I know that diabetes can damage the small blood vessels which then cause a hardening of the arteries which in turn can lead to severe heart issues. We had seen swelling in mom's ankles for a long time now, a sign that the kidneys are not able to get rid of the excess fluids in the body.

Mom will have to understand that the kidneys are near complete failure, and that there is no turning back now. There will be anger and apprehension, but we have to overcome it, and we will as a family.

Dear Reader

Thank you for joining us on the journey that has unfolded. We have lived the lives of Mrs. Murray, a kidney patient, her professional as well as family caregivers, Janice and Sarah, and other support people such as Ben and Geoff, each one bringing to us a dose of emotional as well as intellectual sharing.

Geoff, supervisor, and Janice, Certified Nursing Assistant (CNA), gave us a detailed idea of what is available out there in terms of trained help for people in need. We learned how much it costs to have help like that, how readily available it is, and what the CNAs do for a patient. We also learned that one can cut down on the costs of such caregivers by hiring directly or privately, with the potential pitfalls that it entails.

Naturally, not every professional caregiver is as good and as devoted as Janice, and while the daughter's love can be a constant in care giving, the same cannot always be said about hired caregivers.

At any rate, we saw how people may not be able to afford the high cost of hiring a caregiver, whether privately or through an agency, which explains how come the vast majority of aging Americans are looked after within the confines of the family.

On several occasions "respite care" came into play, whenever Ben came to town, relieving both Sarah and Janice, as well as when Mrs. Murray went to stay at a facility. The truth is that respite care is the motor that keeps many caregiving arrangements going, and without respite care, the caregivers would suffer dramatic bouts of burnout and depression.

We learned a lot about the kidneys, how they work, and how they get distressed, the risk factors that exacerbate them, and the remedies that medicine offers. Mrs. Murray exemplified someone who fell prey to a vicious cycle comprising diseased kidneys, anemia, diabetes, hypertension, fatigue and depression.

When the various options presented themselves, the family chose to take the path of nocturnal (meaning at night) home hemodialysis (HHD). Once Mrs. Murray's GFR fell below 30, and kidney failure was imminent, many things happened simultaneously, and Sarah's and Ben's lives were turned upside down. They had to let Janice go, move mom's belongings to Sarah's home, paint and get ready their mother's home for going on the market, place mom in a short-term facility, and get educated on HHD.

EPILOGUE

Even though Mrs. Murray was at a rough patch during her time in Stage 4 and 5 kidney failure, it's natural as the toxins build up in the blood for the patient to feel worse. At that point, dialysis can only make you feel better because it begins the process of getting your body back to some sort of normalcy. Dialysis takes some time to get used to – whether it's peritoneal dialysis or hemodialysis. In the case of home hemodialysis, once starting on dialysis there is a required amount of training. Sarah has little to be worried about.

People start at the in-center dialysis, but are also started on the training program. This program can take 4-6 weeks, but at the end of the training you are able to do all the necessary steps required to successfully perform dialysis at home. And you always have a person to call at the center to ask questions or get help. All it takes is a willing person and some patience. In Mrs. Murray's case, the 6 weeks of in center dialysis allowed her to get to normal levels of creatinine and BUN blood levels. This made it easier and more comfortable for her to start on home hemo. It seems to help with the insomnia as well by doing nocturnal dialysis, and that appears to be improving the depression.

Mrs. Murray also has a social worker who talks to her and provides some mental health relief for both Sarah and Mrs. Murray by coordinating care for them and providing for their needs. The intrusion is not as bad as Sarah had been concerned about – except for storing the hemodialysis solution. Also, to help with the stress and emotional roller coaster that sometimes happens, Sarah has begun using aromatherapy at dialysis time. She started simply with lavender to calm the environment, and has added some other scents when her mom seems to be agitated. Combining that with gentle reflexology massage using creams that have some essential oils added makes the dialysis time more comfortable. But Mrs. Murray is also becoming more engaged in her care and perks up when Janice visits.

One of the downfalls of home hemodialysis is the potential for isolation. At the center, you have people to engage with, but at home you are up to your own devices whether or not you venture out. Sarah has been creative about finding ways to get her mom to interact. She started by calling Meals on Wheels at the suggestion of her social worker. They come to the house a couple times a week and bring a healthy meal for Mrs. Murray. This alleviates a little of the burden on

Sarah for cooking, and gives her mom some variety. She also checked out the local senior center, and does her weekly errands during times her mom can visit and play bingo or do other activities. The best part is her mom is getting back into her previously fun and favorite activity of quilting. At the senior center they have a quilting group and they are making quilts for the Linus project. (An organization that makes blankets for kids in need to provide security in time of need - www.projectlinus.org) Sarah can get some needed time to work on her tasks for the family, and her mom is making friends. It's not perfect, but she's doing well.

There are always bumps in the road, but the good part of home hemodialysis is the ability to travel. Sarah is planning a trip to Ben's house this summer with her mom and family. She is also investigating ways to allow her mom to travel and utilize an in-center dialysis unit during her travels. Of course, Medicare insurance is one of the things that must be managed in the US, and Sarah is learning a lot about that as well. The family feels like it has been the right decision to go down the road they have, even if it is difficult at times.

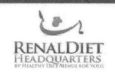

AROMATHERAPY FOR THE CKD PATIENT & CAREGIVER

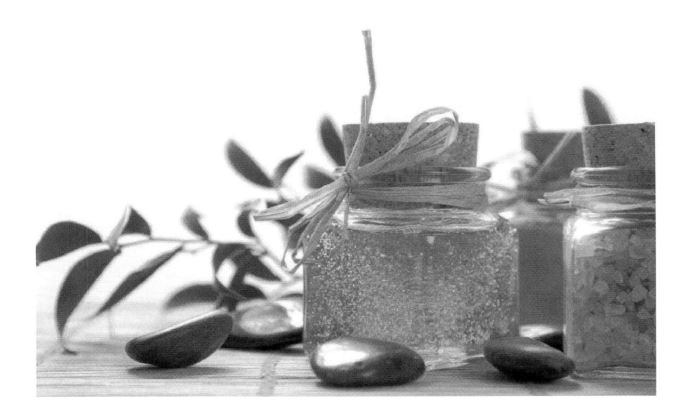

INTRODUCTION TO AROMATHERAPY

When any part of the body dysfunctions it can be terrifying not only for the sufferer but also their loved ones too. With kidney dysfunction, the problems are even more tangible with the introduction of dialysis. Aromatherapy can help.

This book takes you step by step through the challenges and opportunities essential oils present. From soothing infections to calming fractious tensions, it covers all the holistic aspects of healing for kidney patients.

Set out in three parts it provides an in-depth introduction into how aromatherapy and essential oils are used to heal. It assesses the spiritual and emotional dimension of the illness and how these can alter through treatment.

The essential oils section gives insights not only into the outward symptoms of the disease but also how the caregiver can help their days go a little more easily too.

So, without further ado….

Let's investigate how to use aromatherapy for kidney failure.

What is Aromatherapy?

Aromatherapy is a holistic approach to healing using plant essences. The therapist heals not only the physical body, but the emotional and sometimes spiritual disturbances. Even though it can be a curative medicine, legally it can only be termed as giving relief. Essential oils can heal many diseases but in the case of kidney disease the necrotic tissue cannot be repaired. They can however alleviate many of the symptoms which present themselves such as muscle pains, soreness and fatigue as well as helping to guard against threats of infection.

It is important right at the beginning of this book to state aromatherapy is a *complementary medicine*, not as some people state, an alternative medicine. Therapists train for 2 years at the most - as opposed to a medical practitioner who studies for the seven or more years to be qualified. Aromatherapy is effective to support and complement medical advice and never to replace it.

The oils used also complement other therapies and so throughout the book there is reference to acupressure, reflexology and other therapies to bring about incredible relief and healing.

What are Essential Oils?

Essential oils are the concentrated essences of plants containing many healing properties. Some come from flowers, others from woods and barks. Not all plants give up their essences readily so many different methods are used for extracting the oils.

A process you may recognize, distillation, is also used for making whiskey! The oils extracted by distillation are considered to be the only "true essential oils". Aromatherapists use distilled oils, as well as absolutes (oils which are extracted using a solvent) and macerations (plant matter is steeped in vegetable oil to transfer the oil) to heal. To distill an essential oil, plant matter is gathered up into a still and steam is purged through it at a very high pressure. The essential oil molecules vaporize. The steam is captured and cooled leaving behind water with the essential oil floating on the surface.

This floral water or hydrosol can also be used in aromatherapy as it contains very dilute quantities of the oil. These are useful for refreshing skin toners.

How they affect the physical body

In some ways aromatherapy is a misnomer, because it implies smelling the oil will make the body better. This is only part of the truth.

The oils can enter the body in two ways, via the nose (sinuses) and through the skin. (Actually they can also enter by mouth however ***it is not recommended any essential oils be taken orally. They taste dreadful and some can be highly irritating or toxic.***)

When essential oils vaporize, they release a scent, and their healing molecules are liberated. They travel up the nose, along the olfactory nerve to a part of the brain called the limbic system which controls emotions, learning, spatial awareness and memory. From there they can access any part of the brain to trigger changes.

The molecules are a very small and able to penetrate the skin. Just as liquid comes out of your skin when we perspire, so oils can enter into the body through the skin. Once in the body they circulate via the blood stream and can access any of the organs which we want to heal.

What is interesting is unlike the doctor's traditional medicine, essential oils do not have side effects, only main effects. An oil may be uplifting, help skin conditions, be laxative, lower blood pressure and also reduces allergic reactions. While you may choose it to put a spring back in your step or guard against hay fever, you may also find yourself spending more time on the toilet too!

This is covered in more depth in the section about holistic healing but for now, suffice it to say this not only makes them very safe but also means one oil can affect many changes at the same time. For example: Camomile is soothing to the skin and muscles, but it is also calming and can alleviate stomach upsets too.

If you are skeptical, try this little experiment to prove it to you:

Take a clove of garlic. Rub it liberally on the soles of your feet. It will take 20 minutes for the garlic oil to fully permeate through the skin and circulate through the blood stream. After 30 minutes ask someone to smell your breath. The familiar pungent smell will be as strong as having eaten garlic cloves 5 minutes before.

This has very useful implications. Since the oils move through the body, you can apply them anywhere on the body and they will flow where they need to go. Those patients focused on using creams and lotions as a method of application can manage their entire care simply by applying to the inside of the wrist (where the blue veins indicate good blood supply). The essential oils will be absorbed and work well within a small amount of time.

Logic dictates the further the application from the affected part, the weaker the effect. In the case of essential oils, this is not the case. They can be applied close to the affected area or wherever is most convenient, and either placement will yield results. Using creams and lotions means oils can be administered often, in small amounts, and easily. This is an extremely effective method of treatment.

The Blood Brain Barrier

The benefit of the oils comes from the chemical constituents contained within them, and one of those is called a terpene. All helpful elements in the oils have their own properties from being astringent to the skin to being uplifting and relaxing, but some are extremely potent.

Terpenes can be broken down even further and a subset called **sesquiterpenes** exists in the essential oils of most plants. These are the magical ingredients because we now know they are one of the only chemicals which can pass through the blood brain barrier. This discovery has been an amazing breakthrough for science enabling the development of drugs which could herald the end of such diseases as Parkinson's in later generations.

Essential oils and our emotions

The sinus tracts contain the only nerves in the body that go directly to the brain; all others travel via the spinal column. This mean the route to the limbic system through the sinuses is incredibly fast, as quick as five minutes in some people.

Of course this is useful to cheer people up, but it also has more deep routed implications. Research shows that when inhaled, Melissa and lavender oils can help cognition and aggressive behavior in dementia sufferers and rose oil helps to treat trauma from PTSD.

Initially this may seem of no use to you or your family member, but as the oils start to heal you may find new emotions come to the surface. Frustration and anger as well as feelings of hopelessness are common in kidney patients and nearer the end, fear. These feelings are helped a great deal by essential oils. You will find your choices of oils change as you adapt to the needs of your loved one. Don't forget, the oils will affect you as well.

METHODS OF APPLICATION

There are many ways to apply oils and you will find some more suitable than others. The common factor is in all cases the oils must be diluted in some way. Creams and lotions can be used, and of course in the instance of bathing, the water dilutes them.

Often use is intuitive. Once you understand what each oil can do you will see ways in which it can be well integrated.

For example, you might have a wood burning stove. Each evening you could place a metal bowl on top of the stove filled with water, or heat a pan of water gently on the stovetop, and add a drop of lavender and one of rosewood to keep the atmosphere calm and focused on the evening's work. You will discover the same flexibility of aromatherapy as you start to understand your oils.

HOW MUCH TO USE

If you remember nothing else from this book, remember this. When it comes to essential oils *less is more*. There are two main reasons for this and then one specific to kidney function.

First, these oils are incredibly potent. They are capable of healing with one drop, two if really desperate. The body takes what it needs and it sends the rest away to be excreted as waste. Using any more than 2 drops of oil in a preparation is a waste of resources.

Which brings me to my second point: essential oils are expensive. Some of them exorbitant even. (There are good reasons for this from production costs to rarity of plants.) Being frugal with your oils means you will have a resource to draw on for a long time to come.

For kidney patients though, we need to expand on the first point further. When oils are excreted, they are filtered through the kidneys. It is imperative you do not put excess pressure on the kidneys by using too much oil. Over stimulation is a clear hazard for those not adhering to usage guidelines.

Massage

Massage is a very effective method if you have the time and the access to the patient areas that are necessary to place the oils. While the oils absorb through the skin the muscles are warmed and relaxed by the massage. Emotionally, it is soothing and to some people just being touched is extremely therapeutic. Circulation is improved a great deal by massage. This is recommended if the sufferer is struggling to stay warm. This is also the perfect way to get access to valuable reflexology points to stimulate kidney function too.

A full body massage is lovely but not necessary. It could just as easily be a hand, foot or back massage. Remember, the oils work regardless of where they are applied on the body as long as they are absorbed.

Massage oil blending ratios

Use no more than 8 drops of oil in total in 25 mls (1 floz) of oil (2 teaspoons is ample for one massage). If you choose to make a 100mls (4 fl oz) at a time, work to a dilution of no more than 40 drops total. For any individual oil make sure there are no more than 2 drops in a mix.

Essential oils need to be diluted in a carrier oil. There are many of these on the market, each with their own benefits. Simple sunflower oil is a lovely fine oil, olive oil is far thicker and heavier. Borage oil is an excellent base oil for treating stress. There are no hard and fast rules. Experiment to find which ones you like to use best.

Creams and lotions

Creams and lotions are readily available for use. This is the perfect way to administer essential oils using just a small amount and applying often. By putting just a few drops into a readymade lotion you can apply the oils as often as necessary with no need to undress. Just make sure to mix well to ensure even distribution of the oil.

Providing your mix is in a dark colored glass bottle, your blend should keep well for around 5 months.

Creams and Lotions Blending Ratios

Very similar to blending the massage oils, if you choose to make a 100mls (4 fl oz) at a time, work to a dilution of no more than 40 drops total. For any individual oil no more than 2 drops in a mixture of lotion.

Apply a small dab of cream each day. Just enough to cover the pad on the end of your finger

Baths

My favorite application, especially after a long day, is a bath. The warmth of the water opens the pores so the oils can penetrate very easily. Here's a fact for your next dinner party...there are *1,000,000 pores per square inch of skin* making it very easy for oils to absorb. It also softens skin and supports the muscles.

The perfect way to enjoy this kind of luxury is to draw your bath very warm, put your oils in and shut the door. Wait for about 10 minutes to allow the oil molecules to fill your bathroom. Inhaling the gentle scents is incredibly therapeutic and it feels like heaven! Just be careful you check the water temperature before you dip your toe!

Bath Blending Ratios
In a bath of warm water use between 5- 10 drops of oil in total.

Compresses and poultices

A compress or poultice is simply a pad, towel, or wash cloth that is soaked with some essential oil and placed over the affected area.

These play a big part in kidney therapy and in any conditions where there is toxicity or inflammation

They are very simple and effective, but also very relaxing.

We use two types of compresses (also called poultices, packs or pads), hot to open the pores and cold to close them.

To make a hot compress simply fill a small bowl with warm water and add 2 drops of oil. Soak an old piece of cotton towel in the water (Use old towels and washcloths or old baby sheets, dependent on how much is needed) then wring it out well. Do not use boiling water or you will scald the skin.

For a cold compress, the process is the same, except you use cool water instead.

By alternating hot and cold compresses (5 mins each) you can achieve the effect of drawing out deep rooted toxins and open the pores of your skin.

Be aware the tissue salts you draw out will rot the cloth. Wash them out immediately.

Essential oil compresses
Use 5-10 drops in a small bowl of water. Apply the compress to any affected part: For example: forehead for headache or pelvis for urinary infection

Castor Oil Packs
These are same principle as a compress or poultice but take longer.

There is a video which shows you how to prepare and use these:

http://www.renaldiethq.com/go/castoroilpack

THESE ALSO STAIN VERY BADLY SO ALWAYS COVER YOUR BED, CLOTHING AND CHAIRS WELL.

Take a large cotton cloth. It will need to be big enough to cover from the base of your rib cage down to your groin when it has been folded into thirds.

Saturate it with castor oil and then wring it out to avoid dripping. Fold into thirds.

Cover your abdomen from sternum to groin ensuring you cover your lymph nodes.

Cover the towel with grease proof paper or plastic sheet to confine the oil then place a warm water bottle or heating pad on top to heat the oil.

The optimum time to leave the pack is 2 hours but frankly you need a very good book to sustain that. Leave it on for at least 30 minutes.

Evaporators
In effect this is the same as the wood stove trick on a smaller scale. An evaporator or diffuser relies on heat to be applied to the warm oil to allow it to diffuse into the atmosphere. Electric ones are available, as are ones where you place a candle beneath. A bowl of warm water placed on top of the radiator also does the trick.

How much oil to use:
One drop is all that is required to influence the emotions. Any more than that can smell sickly. You may even find you cannot smell the oil when you are in the room

with it. Walk back in after a few minutes and you will notice a big change in your perception. Incidentally, you don't have to be able to smell it for it to be working.

HOMEOPATHIC DOSES

Since the kidneys are in such a weakened state from chronic kidney disease, some of the most powerful oils may be too much for them to cope with. Juniper shifts so much debris it would only put more pressure on the kidneys.

In this case, we use what is called a homeopathic dose. That is $1/15^{th}$ of a drop. It sounds complicated to create but it is not.

Take a carrier oil such as sunflower oil and count out 14 drops (you can find a very useful dropper pipette for this). Add to it one drop of essential oil. Then use one drop of the mix.

Using essential oils on reflexology and acupressure points

Reflexology is an in depth subject and so is covered in a separate book. Incorporating this into your treatment, though, more than doubles the efficacy of the essential oils. Simply massaging the oils over the specific reflexology points introduces them to the kidney meridian.

ACCUPRESSURE POINTS

In Chinese medicine, acupressure and acupuncture is used to stimulate Qi, the living force energy, to run more freely. Blockages in the flow create dis-ease in the organs. These blockages are painful to the touch and can be "emptied" by applying pressure to the points. Use your thumb or a knuckle in circular motions. Be gentle, these points can send patients through the roof; they can be very painful.

Consider integrating these into your treatments. Be careful not to over stimulate the points. Twice a week for twenty minutes is a good balance.

The kidney meridian runs from head to toe down the front of the body and acupressure points are located along it. It runs down the right side of the body down the ribs, down the right hand line of the center of the body, down the inside of the lower leg to the feet.

Human body meridians

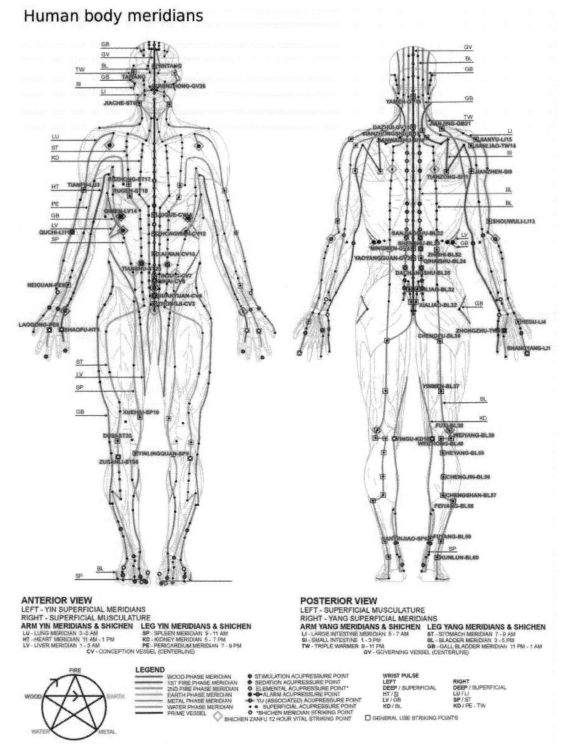

(From Wikipedia.org: http://en.wikipedia.org/wiki/Meridian_(Chinese_medicine))

The leg points are the easiest to access:

The first is on the inside of the calf, aligned with the rear of the knee.

The next three are in three quarters down the calf muscle.

There are four circling the ankle.

Then there are reflex points on the sole.

Reflexology points

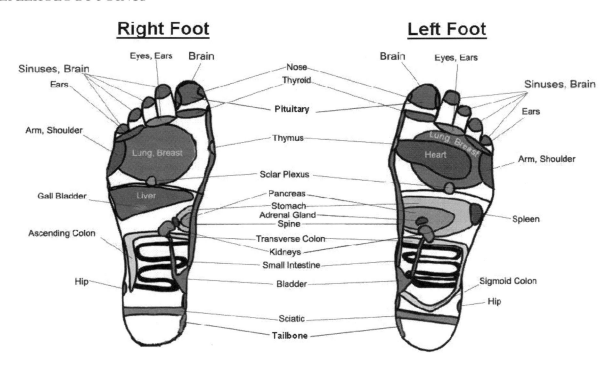

On the soles of the feet, there is a point corresponding to each kidney. Imagine drawing a vertical line from the toes to the heel. Note the halfway point. Now horizontally bisect the halfway mark on the vertical so your foot is divided into four.

On your left foot the upper left quadrant, right next to the crossed lines, relates to the left kidney. The upper right on your right foot relates to the other.

This point is located very close to the acupressure point "Gushing spring" which is used to induce labor, so please do not stimulate these points if you are pregnant.

Holistic Healing

The book opens saying aromatherapy is a holistic therapy, but what does that mean? Well, in fact, it has two references.

The whole

The first, in terms of aromatherapy, is the entire oil of the plant must be used. If you trace the history of plant medicine it will take you back as far as the Ancient Egyptians who used Frankincense to embalm their mummies.

It developed over thousands of years until it reached the 19th Century. Then as the Age of Reason took hold, scientist's left plants behind and begin to make new drugs. Some plants though were too important to ignore and so they learned how to isolate active ingredients to synthesize them. Some you will recognize: valerian was split to make valium, fox gloves were used to make the heart medicine digitalis, and opium poppies give us morphine.

Can you spot the trend? Addiction. The worst of all side effects when only part of the plant is used.

Maintaining the unity of the essential oil components ensure the medicine has no side effects, only many main effects.

The connection between the mind, body and spirit

A holistic medicine practitioner will look at illness as a whole. In other words, where the medical doctor will treat a symptom, holistic medicine tries to work out where the illness originates from. They look at each person as three entities in one. The patient's mind, their body and their spirit, that which is quintessentially you.

Complementary medicine does not look at illness per se, but instead at dis-ease. Notice the hyphenated word. We say the patient is not at ease, they are dis-eased. In fact we say the spirit is diseased and this has evolved through the mind and into the physical body.

So how does it do this?

The aura and chakras

Around the physical body exists subtle bodies. First is an electromagnetic field and then around this, seven layers of energy called the aura. The aura is the seat of the spirit.

It acts as a barometer for the emotions and also for health. You may have seen pictures of the aura taken with kirlian photography, it shows how the colors change from person to person, but actually they change from moment to moment as our moods and health change. For anyone who doubts this, go ahead and walk quietly up behind someone on an escalator. When you permeate their "personal space" they will automatically step forward without even realizing you are there. They will sense you move into their auric field.

The aura connects to our physical body via the chakras. Yoga diagrams demonstrate the 7 major chakras, but there in fact many more. These go through the physical body from front to the back and emanate through the aura.

The chakras open and close as wheels of energy. They rotate in a clockwise direction and vitalize the organs of the body as they run through them.

They connect emotional or spiritual disturbances with the spiritual body. The hypothalamus also connects on a more tangible level.

The following diagram highlights information about the chakras.

THE 7 MAIN CHAKRAS ARE:

	Color	Emotions	Physical
Crown Located at the top of the head.	Purple	Empathy Compassion	Brain Head Nervous System Pineal Gland
Brow (Or Pineal)	Indigo	The third eye Perception Intuition True motivations	Forehead Caritoid Plexus
Throat Located at the base of the throat	Blue	Communication. The sense of giving and getting what you want and need and expressing this.	Neck Throat Arms Hands Brachial & Cervical Plexus
Heart	Green	Love Openness and relating Separation from love Grief	Heart Blood Circulatory System Lungs Chest area Thymus gland
Solar Plexus	Yellow	Power Control Freedom Ease of being one's self The face we show the world	Skin Liver Spleen Gall bladder Intestines Eyes The face
Sacral	Orange	Relationship between what the body wants and needs With food With Sex Having children Willingness to feel emotions Learning to relate with others Feelings of control by another person	Reproductive system Sexual organs Genito-urinary system Inc Kidneys Lumbar organs Ovaries and Testes Pituitary Gland

		Survival	Nose
Base (or Root)	Red	Survival Trust Relationship with money and wealth Way that one makes one's living Relationship with mother And with Mother Earth To be nourished physically	Nose Lymph system skeleton system Teeth and bones Prostate gland in men Sacral plexus Bladder Elimination system Lower extremities (Legs ,feet, ankles etc)

KIDNEY RELATIONSHIP WITH THE SACRAL CHAKRA

You will notice that the sacral chakra governs the kidneys. You may also recognize some of the emotions connected with it.

In times of emotional imbalance or strong emotions, it will throw the chakra out of balance. It may jar it open, or shut it tight. When this happens, the organs can no longer be vitalized correctly. The easiest example to demonstrate this is grief. It jars the heart chakra open. (Have you ever felt that weird ache in your chest?) The out pouring of grief (heart energy) weakens the physical heart and a person suffers "a broken heart". Oversimplified somewhat, but you get the drift.

DISCERNING THE CHAKRAS

An experiment: to "draw the chakras". This will help you to see them more easily. A chakra specialist uses a crystal pendulum to point this but it can be just as easily done with anything which is heavy at the bottom and will swing like a pendulum; a ring on a chain works well.

Get your partner to lie down on their back and then holding the pendulum about 6 inches from the body. Draw a line, with the pendulum swinging on the vertical, down the center point of their body from head to toe. Periodically the pendulum will stop swinging in a straight line and catch up in a chakra and beginning swinging in a clockwise direction.

In health the chakra will swing the pendulum in a circle. If it whizzes very fast it shows it is jarred open. If there is little swing or it traces an ellipse, the chakra is closed. Oftentimes chakras move out of line too.

Some people use meditation or chakra singing bowls to vitalize the chakras. You also can use essential oils.

Emotional connections with kidneys and sacral chakra

You will recall that essential oils have many main effects. You may find while you are treating the physical aspects of the disease some strange and possibly challenging emotions rear their heads. This is the oils healing the patient in their entirety. Don't worry. Revisit the oils list to tackle any which become difficult. Make sure you give it a little time to process.

Often the emotional disturbance which triggered the physical response may come to the surface. Usually at the beginning of the treatment, the patient may not recognize any of the connections. They can cause arguments as the mind unlocks things they have wanted to say. This expression is vital to allow the body to heal.

There are a myriad of possibilities. In fact, there are as many combinations as there are patients. Armed with this information, watch with a wry smile as you witness the magic you created with your bottle of oil. You can create health as the oils flow and release the patient, and even though you are not healing the kidney disease – the improvement will be obvious.

The hypothalamus – the bridge between mental and physical healing

This little organ is found in the brain and it controls all of the hormones in the body. Based on the emotions the body is exhibiting, it decides what amounts to produce and triggers the organs to do so. Imagine this as a rather "mad" conductor instructing the organs with his baton.

On a physical level this is why you have diarrhea when you are waiting for an exam, or your heart beats faster on meeting a new lover. This is another bridge between emotional and physical dis-ease.

Physical healing

Many of the oils chosen have antiseptic properties which reduce risks of infection.

OILS FOR THE KIDNEYS

The main oils which I feel will best help chronic kidney problems are:

Black pepper
Use this oil in small quantities if a fever spikes from infection. Black pepper oil stimulates the sacral chakra.

Camomile Maroc
This is a calming and soothing oil. Really it should be top of your shopping list. You will see it appear many times in these notes. Most interesting is its direct correlation between the emotional and physical aspects of kidney disease. In her book the Garden of Eden, Jill Bruce says of it:

"Physical: It is very soothing, carminative, anti-inflammatory-antiseptic. Starting to evolve to deal with bacteria or virus carried within the lymphs. There is a connection with kidneys and excretion. Seems to be able to help renal colic.

Mental: It helps people to sink away under their problems. Seems to make problems feel less acute.

Spiritual: Seems to soothe family rows and allows communication to flow between people more easily."

Castor Oil
An extremely cleansing and stimulating oil, castor oil is a maceration rather than an essential oil. It is recommended that castor oil packs be administered for a period of 28 days to draw out as much toxicity is possible. Continuity of this treatment is important as castor oil continues to work for 12 hours after a pack has been used, but then stops working. Do not use in menstruation or if pregnancy is suspected.

Cypress
Cypress is one of the best oils for treating any problem with the genito- urinary tract.

The kidneys play a part in the production of red blood cells and cypress plays a part in helping the body to manufacture these more effectively.

It is quite astringent and very cleansing too. Cypress oil has the capacity to lift your mood or the atmosphere; it is a very happy oil and is particularly good for helping frustration.

Because of its astringent effects, use no more than 2 drops of this in the bath to avoid possible skin irritation.

Fennel (Sweet)
This is a very strong diuretic and it is suggested to use a homeopathic dose. A strong antitoxic fennel very quickly cleanses the entire bodily system including the blood.

Edema is well healed with the oil when used in massage. It is also a very carminative oil which means it not only helps nausea but also flatulence as well. Strongest of all, it gives courage in the face of difficult medical situations.

This oil should be avoided by patients with epilepsy. Instead replace with juniper, also in a homeopathic dose.

Frankincense
This is a very cleansing oil and will help the kidneys but its best effects fall in a more spiritual plane. A great instiller of confidence frankincense deals with the stubbornness which comes with the acknowledgement of disease. When you hear, "What has God done for me?" Grab the frankincense.

Geranium
This lovely oil is an overall tonic. It invigorates and balances every system in the body. It is sedative and relaxing. On days which are very hard, put 5 drops in the bath and feel the weight of the world just drift away.

Ginger
This is a favorite oil to use when patients are struggling with some sort of moisture, whether that is urination (or in deed lack of it), diarrhea or even sweating. It has anticoagulant properties, so avoid use if you are taking blood thinners.

Aching joints, rheumatism and arthritis all feel relief from ginger. It is used for muscle spasms. It is a very warming oil, and when using it, the heat travels upwards, so massage the feet for the best effect. It is an excellent guard against infection.

Lastly, its stimulating effects are useful if libido begins to wane.

Again...watch dosage; no more than 2 drops in any application to avoid skin irritation.

Jasmine
This oil is used for its sexual dimension as it is a very powerful aphrodisiac, helping to remove psychological blocks. It is especially helpful to men. It is however an expensive oil and you may find a combination of nutmeg and geranium to be as effective.

Juniper
This is another oil for you to use in a homeopathic dose. Juniper cleanses the joints of built up uric acid which causes aches and pains. Again this vibrates on orange (the sacral chakra) and is also very involved emotionally in setting the record straight.

Lavender
Lavender is, without doubt, the most efficacious oil in the box.

It is soothing and relieves pain. It is emotionally calming and antiseptic.

There are many chemotypes of this oil. The most effective will be *Lavendula angustifolia* which psychologically is a very helpful oil for guiding the caregiver to understand the patients needs.

Lemon
Lemon is a very strong antiseptic so do not use this oil in the bath as it will irritate the skin.

It is a valuable aid to healing infection as it encourages production of leucocytes which are the antibodies which raise immunity. It encourages appetite and raises blood pressure.

Mandarin
This is the most important oil for treating both exhaustion and fatigue as it stimulates and supports the adrenal glands. These secrete adrenaline when we are stressed and over time become depleted. Every physiological problem resulting from stress is helped by mandarin.

It is a tonic to the kidneys and also promotes harmonious atmospheres when used in an evaporator.

Marjoram
As it works on the central nervous system, marjoram is the best oil for healing insomnia. Use no more than one drop in a treatment as larger amounts can be intoxicating

Muscle spasms, aches and pains are all alleviated using marjoram.

Another effect to be aware of is its ability to reduce libido.

Nutmeg
Use one drop only of this very stimulating oil in any treatment. It is a superb companion with mandarin as it stimulates the pituitary gland in harmony with mandarin's effect on the adrenals. Together these help the external symptoms of stress such as irritability, insomnia, impotence and loss of sexual appetite.

It stimulates hunger. Warming the joints and encouraging better blood circulation it is an excellent oil to add into muscle rubs and massage oils.

Patchouli
Delicious and heady patchouli is relaxing, restorative and ultra sexy! It is an oil which does not appeal to everyone, so check that you both like the fragrance before "the big event."

Rose
Rose is the gentlest and most effective healer of anything pertaining to reproduction. It is included here for its subtleness in seduction. Relationships can be tested when there is a chronic illness. This oil is about love and sex, rather than lust.

Rosemary
This is a remarkable oil for dealing with pain, especially in the joints and particularly nerve pain. Do not use if you have high blood pressure or epilepsy.

Always use this oil in any condition where there is a loss of function (as in kidney) for its stimulating effects. It stimulates appetite and is the most invigorating of all essential oils.

Emotionally it has a harsh edge to it. If conversations become spiteful, burn some lavender to smooth them down.

Spikenard

A very ancient oil, spikenard is blue. It's color comes from the chemical constituent azulene which is, in effect, a liquid anesthetic. This is an expensive oil but it is useful if a condition becomes very acute. Chronic pain and terrible insomnia are both helped by spikenard. It is also antibacterial.

Tea tree

This is the king of all anti bacterial and antiseptics. It also vibrates on the colour orange which is also the vibration of the sacral chakra. This is a very important oil to use for chronic kidney disease sufferers.

Ylang ylang

This is oil is a balancing oil. If the blood pressure is too high or low, it will settle it. It is an aphrodisiac because it relaxes the mind and body so much. To some degree it is antiseptic, but there are better oils to use for this effect.

OILS WHICH SHOULD BE AVOIDED IN CHRONIC KIDNEY DISEASE ARE:
You may see the following essential oils recommended for kidney complaints; however, once a patient has reached the need for dialysis they are too weakened to cope with these rigorous and potent oils.

Avoid: **Aloe, Buckthorn, Camphor, Capsicum, Cascara, Chapparal, Cinnamon, Comfrey, Dandelion, Ephedra, Licorice, Mate, Nettle, Noni Juice, Pennyroyal, Rhubarb, Sassafras, Segrada, Senna**

The following have anticoagulant properties and should be avoided if you are taking blood thinners: Ginger, Gingko Biloba, Garlic, Ginseng, Feverfew

HELPING THE PHYSICAL SYMPTOMS BROUGHT ON BY CHRONIC KIDNEY DISEASE

Itchy skin
Camomile, Lavender

Staphylococcal infections
Tea Tree, ginger and cypress.

Low blood pressure
Lavender, lemon, marjoram, ylang ylang

Fatigue and tiredness
Mandarin, basil, cypress, lavender, marjoram, rosemary, nutmeg

Difficulties falling asleep (insomnia) or staying asleep
Lavender, camomile, spikenard

Achiness, Bone and Joint pain
Juniper – homeopathic dose *(see page 12)*, Lavender, Cypress, Black pepper, Rosemary – especially with nerve pain, Geranium

Loss of libido (sex drive)
Ylang ylang, Patchouli, Rose, Jasmine

Also marjoram can be of use in that it reduces libido in the other party. Sometimes healing is all about compromise.

OILS FOR THE EMOTIONS

Anger
Rose, camomile, lavender, geranium, melissa

Anxiety
Lavender, camomile, marjoram, geranium

Depression
Melissa, bergamot, ginger, rose

Fear
Angelica (of dying), marjoram, camomile

Frustration
Thyme, geranium, bergamot

Stress

To soothe: Lavender, camomile, geranium, rose

To support the adrenals: Mandarin.

OILS TO BALANCE THE SACRAL CHAKRA (ASSOCIATED WITH THE KIDNEYS)
Black pepper, bulgarian lavender, juniper, mandarin, neroli (orange blossom), naiouli, palma rosa, rose, spearmint, ylang ylang

OILS FOR THE CAREGIVER

Melissa and bergamot will put a spring back in your step and geranium will melt the day away but sometimes that is not enough.

Thyme is a good oil to use if you are feeling you are getting no recognition for what you are doing. It gives an understanding of your own self worth.

Always try to integrate mandarin into your own treatments to avoid exhaustion.

CONTRAINDICATIONS AND SAFETY DATA

Reminder: There are no side effects from essential oils, only main effects. This is a very positive thing but it can also have its drawbacks.

In some cases, there may be irritation from essential oils. If this occurs, rinse well with copious amounts of water.

It is probably obvious, but avoidance of any possible allergens is important. For instance, nut allergies will most likely be triggered by nutmeg oil.

Do not take essential oils internally. If they are swallowed, call your local poison control center hotline and explain to them what you consumed. Take the oil bottle with you to the emergency room. The doctor can then assess any possible damage and decide treatment accordingly.

PREGNANCY

This is a delicate time in a mother's life, but even more so for an unborn child. There is little research to tell us how the oils affect a fetus. What we do know is they continue to affect the internal physiology of the mother. They can raise blood pressure, or in many cases instruct the uterus to contract...which in early pregnancy results in miscarriage.

As a guideline then, there are virtually no oils which should be used by women before 12 weeks have elapsed.

The following essential oils should be avoided during the first **16** weeks:

Angelica, Black Pepper, Clove, Cypress, Eucalyptus, Ginger, Helichrysum, Marjoram, Myrrh, Nutmeg, Oregano, Peppermint, Roman Chamomile, Basil, Cinnamon Bark, Lemongrass, Rosemary, Thyme, Vetiver, White Fir.

Myrrh, Rose, Jasmine and Clary sage all contract the uterus. Do not use during pregnancy. If you are the caregiver, remember you will be affected by the oils as well and act accordingly.

Oils to be avoided entirely in pregnancy are tarragon, valerian, wintergreen, parsley leaf, penny royal and sage.

Lactation
Essential oils can be tasted in breast milk and so you may find it puts baby off feeding. Carrot Seed Oil will enhance milk flow, Geranium helps soothe engorged breasts, and Marigold can heal cracked nipples. All others should be used with care.

If baby stops feeding, stop using oils for a day and see what happens.

Menstruation
Heavy bleeding and menstrual problems are generally helped using essential oils but avoid using castor oil packs during the week of your period to avoid bleeding too heavily.

High blood pressure
Avoid hyssop, rosemary, sage and thyme in cases of high blood pressure. Oils which are beneficial however are: clary sage, marjoram, melissa, geranium and ylang ylang.

Epilepsy
Some oils contain what we call neurotoxins and can bring on seizures in epilepsy suffers. Avoid camphor, rosemary, spike lavender *(see notes on chemotypes on page 25)* and tarragon.

Buying essential oils

Over the last 30 years aromatherapy has undergone many changes from fringe crank medicine to mainstream healing. In light of this, supply of essential oils has changed. In the early '80's, oils could only be obtained from very specialist suppliers but as knowledge began to pervade the public consciousness they became more and more available.

In the '90s every supermarket shelf touted some wonder shampoo with tea tree and essential oils were available in equal readiness.

Now the main shopping mall is found on the information super highway and it is easier than ever to get your hands on a new bottle of oil.

But how do you know which are the good sellers and which are the bad?

Correct labeling

Always look to see the Latin name of the plant is given as well as the English. Good suppliers will know to write the first name capitalized but not the second so: *Lavendula latifolia.*

You should also be able to read the country of origin and also the purity of the oil. Ideally you want to see 100% pure essential oil, but that is not always the case as some oils may be "cut" with others. This need not necessarily be a bad thing. Lemon balm for instance is often labeled Melissa (Type) rather than Melissa (True). This means it has been cut with lemon verbena oil to make it go further. Melissa officinalis has a yield of less than 0.033% oil from plant matter so it costs a huge amount of money to produce it. As it is therapeutically such an important oil, it makes it accessible at a much more reasonable price.

Labels should show what has been used to dilute the oils. Often rose oil may be in sunflower oil for example. This is fine, it is just considerably weaker.

When buying oils, head for the health food store first. They will usually have many of the more popular oils in stock. For more unusual ones, go to Amazon and specialist websites too.

A good indicator is to look at the write ups they have given the oils. How in depth are they? Do they seem to have a good grasp of their stock and do they explain any possible dangers of use? If so then these should be top of your list. Here are three excellent ones to give you a head start.

http://www.essentialoils.co.za/

https://www.mountainroseherbs.com/

http://www.amphora-aromatics.com/

CHEMOTYPES

There are often many different subspecies of the same plant. There are yellow roses, climbers and bushes. Every single one creates a slightly different oil. We call these chemotypes. Some chemotypes of oil work differently from others and in some cases this can cause a safety issue.

There are several subspecies of lavender, some with white flowers, some with pretty pink tufts. As with any plant they adapt to the environment in which they grow. They absorb toxicity from their surroundings, from the soil and from the air. It affects the both the quality and the properties of the oils.

There are many chemotypes of lavender oil. Alpine lavender is extremely pure and gentle, whereas Croation Lavender still has the harshness of war to it. It is no lesser oil, it simply heals in a different way…in fact it has evolved to remove petrochemicals from the liver. It is an important oil for a different reason.

There are two chemotypes of lavender to avoid. *Lavendula latifolia* also called Spike Lavender, which can be neurotoxic and also cause muscle cramps. *Lavendula stoechas* is an abortive and should be avoided in pregnancy.

OXIDATION

Because the oils are taken from living plants, essential oils do have a shelf life. Some are longer than others. Those taken from citrus oils are very short. Your bottle will start to lose its effectiveness after about six months. Others will last longer, up to even ten years.

If the oil starts to smell or look rancid, oxidation is your problem and the oil should be discarded.

To prolong the shelf life, follow the storage guidelines.

STORING ESSENTIAL OILS

Oils should be kept in a cool dark place. Always ensure you secure the top of the bottle well to avoid evaporation and also oxidation.

Most important: Keep out of reach of children.

BIBLIOGRAPHY

The author would like to thank the writers of the following text books and websites for the insights they have given to this research.

Robert Tisserand – The Art of Aromatherapy

Patricia Davis – Aromatherapy an A-Z

Jill Bruce – The Garden of Eden

Dr Jean Valnet – The Practice of Aromatherapy

Valerie Ann Worwood – Aromantics

Natalie Kent – The Mind Body Connections

Consumer Lab: www.consumerlab.com

NSF International Quality Label: www.nsf.org

USP Verified: www.uspverified.org

National Center for Complementary and Alternative Medicine: http://nccam.nih.gov/

Alternative Medicine Facts: http://www.rosenthal.hs.columbia.edu/CAM.html

Herbal Research Foundation: www.herbs.org

Alternative Medicine Foundation: www.herbmed.org

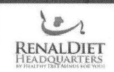

REFLEXOLOGY & RENAL DISEASE

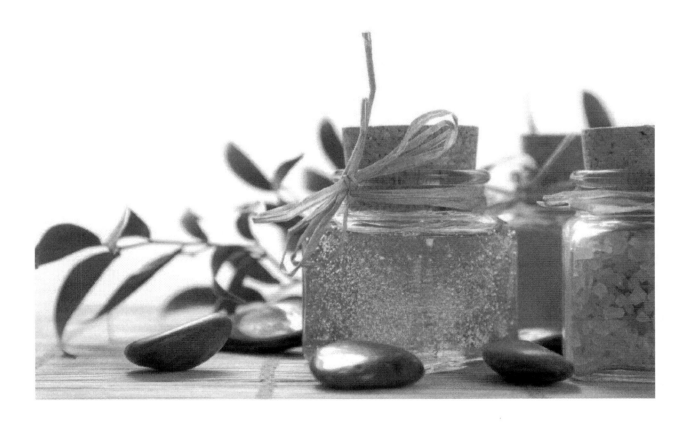

An Overview

If you have a spouse, parent or another loved one going through kidney failure, the strain of the illness must be taking its toll on you as well. In such a situation, you must already be trying out and searching for new techniques and methods that will help the person you care for in getting comfortable during this difficult time. If this is what you are doing, the reflexology treatment is one option you must consider.

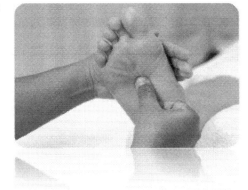

However, before you start to learn the ropes and understand this successful treatment, you must consult a doctor or practitioner since kidney failure and other serious diseases need the utmost care and attention. Therefore, even though there is no harm in the reflexology treatment for patients with kidney failure, a doctor should know beforehand about your plans to use this method.

Many people are turning towards this alternative remedy for kidney failure because it has only a few, if any, side effects and is as effective as the cupping therapy (a Chinese alternative medicine where suction is created using heat to mobilize the blood and promote heating), acupuncture (a traditional Chinese treatment where thin needles, heat, pressure or laser is used to correct imbalances in the energy flow), and moxibustion (a traditional Chinese therapy that uses dried mugwort along with acupuncture needles or to burn it on the skin). In addition, reflexology can help you treat serious medical conditions like asthma, diabetes, and even cancer.

Through this booklet, you will discover everything there is to know about the reflexology treatment, starting from what it is and all the way to how you can implement it. Once you have finished reading the last line, you will not only have information about how to provide specific hand and feet massages, but you will also know the theoretical side of this alternative treatment, assuring your loved one that you are giving them what is best for their case.

So, without further delay, move on to the first chapter so that you can understand exactly what reflexology is, how it works and how it can benefit your loved one.

UNDERSTANDING REFLEXOLOGY TREATMENT

Understanding reflexology is essential, especially since most caregivers have a tough time explaining why they need to resort to alternative methods. Therefore, before you can go ahead and explain it to your loved one, you should know every aspect to answer their questions.

DEFINING REFLEXOLOGY

Reflexology uses special finger and hand techniques to apply pressure to specific sensitive areas of the feet, hands and ears. Basically, there are areas in the hands and feet which correspond to organs and systems of the body. By applying pressure onto the right points, reflexology can increase your blood circulation, promote metabolism, and regulate qi (*the Chinese medicine and martial arts term for energy flow or life force*) and blood.

Now the main goal of reflexology is to use specific massage and pressure techniques on the critical points reflexes of the hands or feet and remove any energy blocks that may be there due to reasons like stress, a bad lifestyle or unhealthy diet. As a result, the massages will assist in helping energy currents flow freely and the body will once again return to its harmonious state.

However, in order to ensure the success of reflexology, you should find the primary cause of the problem. This is why anyone using reflexology to get relief from pain or stress must also combine this technique with other forms of treatment. This ensures that reflexology pays off in a shorter time.

HOW IT WORKS

Also referred to as zone therapy, reflexology is based on a concept developed by American physician William Fitzgerald from Hartford, Connecticut. According to this zone system concept, there are ten separate current energy channels that circulate throughout the body. These channels, which are divided equally across both part of the body, flow in longitudinal lines

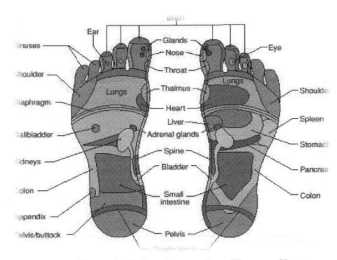

Figure 1 - Reflexology or Zone Therapy Chart

from TaschMar Holistic Health

called zones. Within these zones are the organs and muscles of the body, which are tackled during the reflexology treatment.

When the energy currents that flow through the longitudinal zones accumulate, and build up at specific points, they create what is known as energy blockage. These interrupted points, which are commonly known as energy blocks interrupt the smooth flow of the energy throughout the body or in areas causing pain, disease or disorder.

THE BENEFITS OF REFLEXOLOGY TREATMENT

For decades, reflexology has been applied in the cases of many kidney failure patients. If you read about Traditional Chinese Medicine, you will find that these practices believe that kidney diseases or kidney failure is the result of an imbalance in yin, yang, qi, blood, which is due to wind, cold, heat, damp, dryness, trauma and other such external conditions. Pressure zones that correspond to the kidney function can promote the qi and the circulation of blood in the kidneys, which in turn will help relieve patients' symptoms.

When you properly learn reflexology techniques and discover the various pressure points, you will be able to massage different parts of the feet according to where the lesion or problem is located. However, before you go any further, you need to learn the concept of the meridian system as this is what reflexology depends on. The meridian system is a Chinese medicine belief about the path in which qi flows. The network is divided into two categories:

1. **Jingmai** – Also known as the meridian channels (the lines through which the energy of the body is believed to flow in Chinese medicine), this category contains 12 tendinomuscular meridians (meridians on the surface of the body that protect against the assault of external viruses and bacteria starting from the toe tips and fingertip points), 12 divergent meridians (paths that protect against viruses and bacteria, and used to travel through lymph ducts, Polarity treatment, immune diseases, and movement disorders), 12 principal meridians (meridians in charge of nourishing all the tissue in the body), 8 extraordinary vessels (channels that are irregularly distributed and do not have direct relations with organs) as well as the Huato channel (bilateral points at the lower back).
2. **Luomai** – Known as associated vessels or collaterals, this category consists of 15 major arteries that are linked to the 12 principal meridians.

These are the points through which the energy flows; therefore, when you manipulate them, you will be able to provide relief. When you stimulate the accupoints on the feet, the meridians will be dredged, qi stagnation will be eliminated, and blood circulation will start to flow once again.

Therefore, massaging the specific reflex zones of the kidney, urethra and bladder will help in treating kidney failure, improve the urinary function and kidney operations, and promote the discharge of toxins and wastes from the body of the patient.

Aside from renal failure, reflexology will also help you in solving other symptoms that are associated with chronic kidney disease, including:

- Fatigue
- Sleep Difficulties
- Frequent Urination
- Edema
- Appetite Loss
- Bone or Joint Pain
- Trouble Breathing
- Loss of Sexual Interest
- Itching or Dry Skin
- Edema
- Nausea and Vomiting
- Headaches or Migraines

In fact, there are a large group of people who claim that even though their medicines were not able to bring them a lot of relief for the afore mentioned symptoms, going for long and regular reflexology sessions helped them find balance and joy in their lives.

Before learning more about reflexology and its positive effect on kidney failure, it is important that you know that this alternative medicine technique is a holistic approach. This means that the patient must be involved and willing to work with you during the treatment process. In addition, because reflexology centers on massage and pressure to the reflex areas in the feet and hands, it is crucial that you learn the anatomy of each of these parts. Therefore, you must make sure to have in-depth knowledge about both the hands and the feet.

However, before you invest your time and effort in learning about reflexology, you may want an additional incentive to start learning its techniques. To assure you that you are making the right decision, the following chapter will highlight how successful this alternative technique is.

HOW EFFECTIVE IS REFLEXOLOGY FOR KIDNEY FAILURE

Even though reflexology will not cure the kidney failure that your loved one is going through, it will surely help in easing and even relieving the pain and other symptoms.

Sudmeier et al. (1999) conducted a research study where they used 32 healthy subjects to measure the blood flow of the three major vessels of the kidney, before and after reflexology. The results, which were measured using Doppler sonography, showed that reflexology was effective in increasing the renal blood flow during therapy. This and many other studies have shown that reflexology will help with at least some of the problems that a patient with renal failure is facing.

Another study conducted by Williamson in 2002 showed that both foot massage as well as reflexology helped greatly in reducing anxiety and depression. This is helpful because kidney failure patients can be quite anxious and stressed. If you know how to properly perform reflexology, you will be able to help your patient by easing the anxiety that they are feeling and lend a hand in making them feel relaxed.

27 different and distinctive studies have also shown that there is significant pain reduction in patients who go through a 15-30 minute reflexology session. Some of the diseases with which these studies have been conducted are renal failure, AIDS, chest pain, peripheral neuropathy of diabetes mellitus, and kidney stones.

In other controlled studies, such as the one conducted by Hodgson in 2000, results showed that there was 100% improvement in people who were in the reflexology group for a number of symptoms. Not only were the patients able to improve their nausea and pain, but they also reported improvement in sleep cycles and tiredness.

Now that you know how science and researchers positively view reflexology, you may be more willing to try it or recommend it to your ailing loved one. This means that you are ready to learn the practical aspects of reflexology.

THE REFLEXOLOGY AREA

Even though reflexology is mostly practiced on the hands, feet and ears, the two zones that receive the most attention are the first two. Therefore, this chapter will focus on these to help you provide the best massages to kidney failure patient.

STRUCTURE OF THE FEET AND HANDS

Each foot consists primarily of twenty six bones and thirty three articulations. These bones and articulations are joined together by hundreds of ligaments. The muscles of the feet are very delicate when compared to the hands, the latter which are primarily designed for precise and intricate movements while the muscles of your feet ensure locomotion.

On the other hand, each of your hands and wrists consist of twenty seven bones and tendons altogether. The movement of the thumb is quite important. The general function of the hands will include the power gripping, precision handling, and other such complex operations, but these depend on specialized movements from the thumb, some of which you need to utilize during your reflexology treatment session.

CRUCIAL ZONES

Because modern reflexology works on the basis on zone therapy, it is important that you understand where these ten longitudinal zones lie. Now the ten zones are divided into five zones on each of the side of the body:

Zone One: The first zone extends from the tip of both thumbs until the top of the head and then down through the nostrils to the tip of the big toes.

Zone Two: This zone extends from the very tip of the index finger to the head and down to the tip of the second toes.

Zone Three: The third zone is that from the tip of the second finger to the head and then down to the tip of the third toe.

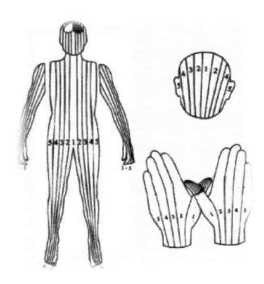

Figure 2 – Crucial Zones from International Institute of Reflexology, France

Zone Four: This zone begins from the tip of the ring fingers to the head and goes down to the tip of the fourth toe.

Zone Five: The final zone starts from the little finger to the head and reaches the end at the tip of the little toe.

Once you know about each of these zones, you can easily map out the body systems, glands and organs which are within the appropriate zones. As shown in the diagram on the right, the kidney (detailed in blue), is located in the arch of the foot, therefore this is the region or zone which you need to focus on.

THINGS TO CONSIDER BEFORE STARTING REFLEXOLOGY

Before you start reflexology techniques and massages, it is important that you know about some of the most important points to consider during the process. Make sure that you think about everything discussed in this chapter so that the reflexology sessions are effective and beneficial for the patient.

ALWAYS CARRY OUT THE WHOLE TREATMENT

Reflexology sessions are usually carried out on both the hands and feet. Even if you are only focusing on the feet, you must avoid doing massages for specific organs or symptoms. Experts suggest that the best way to go is to focus on the entire area and then go back to the reflex points which you want to target, in this case the kidney. This general rule of thumb is applied when you carry out reflexology for the feet, hands, ears or any other areas.

ASK FOR FEEDBACK

Because you are going to be doing the reflexology on someone who has kidney failure, you must take care as these patients are often sensitive to touch. For this reason, it is important that you keep asking them for feedback and ask whether the pressure you are applying is good for them or not. The pressure you add should also be less than you would use on a healthy person because such patients are usually sensitive. After two to three sessions, you will not need to ask the patient about their level of comfort because you will already know the pressure which suits them best.

USE CREAMS AND OILS

Though they should be used in moderation, oils and creams can be used to make it easier for you to move your hands during the sessions. The best way to go is to use the oil when initially starting with the treatment session because this will help the skin absorb the oils as you go forward. However, when using any oils or creams, make sure that the patient is not sensitive or allergic to the ingredients used in making them. If you feel that there is a lot of oil making your hands slip, you can always opt for some talcum powder to absorb the oil. You can add aromatherapy oils to combine the treatments and improve the effects.

CLEAN AND INSPECT

When you are about to begin the reflexology session, it is important that you wipe the surface area with some wet wipes or similar products to clean the foot thoroughly. You can also use slightly perfumed tissues as well as this will help in relaxing the receiver. This will also give you the chance to inspect and detect any problems with the patient's feet which may cause hindrance in your session. Also make sure that the patient's toe nails have been trimmed and cleaned properly so that both you and they do not get hurt during the sessions.

Practice Your Techniques

When trying to provide the best reflexology sessions to your loved one, you must ensure that you first practice the technique on yourself. Use your own foot or hand while learning the methods as this will not only help you get the hang of the procedure, but it will ensure that the patient is not hurt in any way once you start the sessions. Individuals who perform reflexology on their parents or spouses often say that it is best to start practicing at least a month before administering the treatment on others.

People Have Physical Responses to Reflexology

Because you are going to be targeting specific reflex points during the course of your reflexology sessions, it is not uncommon for people to give unintentional physical responses such as burps, coughs and spasms. You must also know that each patient will be different; while some people experience an increase in energy levels, others feel very relaxed and may even say that they have flu like symptoms. However, if these reactions or responses have stopped 24 hours after the treatment session, there is nothing for you to worry about. Moreover, these responses are most evident in patients going through reflexology for the first time since their bodies are adjusting to changes. As time passes, you will note that the reactions will grow less with every session.

Use Relaxing Massages Where Necessary

Relaxing massages and techniques are necessary during a reflexology treatment because they help you alter the pace, change the areas where you are working and keep things light and a little exciting during the sessions. Do not confuse reflexology with massage techniques as the former is used majorly as a treatment method while the latter is suggested for relaxation and ease.

Implementing Reflexology Treatment

Now that you have learned about the crucial aspects of reflexology and renal failure, you are ready to start learning about the treatment and everything you must consider during reflexology.

Duration and Frequency of Reflexology

Where reflexology is concerned, you must ensure that the sessions are neither too long nor too short for the patient. The average time used in reflexology is 30-40 minutes because the results and positive changes are obvious after this time. However, though this is the recommended time, some experts suggest that you shorten the session to 10-20 minutes for patients that are in the end stages of the kidney failure. The time should be adjusted according to the specific illness and the conditions faced by the patient. Start with 10-20 minutes for the first few sessions.

If you have a chronic kidney failure patient, you can give them a massage 2-4 times each week while those who have critical symptoms and conditions can be allowed to give one massage every day. Once again, you must bear in mind that the strength and pace should vary because patients with severe conditions often prefer and find relief when the pace is quicker.

Moreover, the patient should be allowed to drink 10-16 ounces of water half an hour after the reflexology session. This will help in discharging the toxic wastes from the body. However, if the patient is in the final stages of renal failure and is not too fond of drinking water, you can always reduce the amount to 5 ounces. Just make sure that they do drink the water given to them.

Environment

The place or environment where you carry out the reflexology treatment and sessions should be comfortable and have a pleasant surrounding that promotes peace and relaxation. Also remember that the average time lapse between treatments should be three days. However, this number can vary according to the condition and symptoms the patient faces. These two to three days in between the sessions will help the body eliminate the toxins activated through the reflexology sessions.

Moreover, if this is the first time that you are giving your loved one the massage, you must be prepared to answer some of their questions because they may not know what to expect and may even dread the outcomes of the procedure. Therefore, experts suggest that you explain exactly what is going to happen even before you begin so that the patient can be calm and relaxed during the treatment. You must also tell them that it is important that they inform you if they feel any pain when pressure is applied because this will indicate that the energy (qi) is being blocked.

You must also tell them about any possible side effects of the reflexology treatment, such as fatigue, sweating, and an urge to visit the bathroom more often and so on. Also make sure that you know about the medical history of the person who you are performing the reflexology on as this will help you gain insight on their present problem and symptoms. Finally, prior to beginning the actual treatment, you must check out your patient's feet and hands, as their condition will give you a lot of crucial information.

MASSAGE TECHNIQUES
Video to learn techniques: http://www.renaldiethq.com/go/reflexologyvideo

In general, because it is easier to work with a stationary foot or hand as opposed to a moving one, it is recommended that you use one hand to practice the massages, while the other should act as the 'holding' hand to keep the foot in place. Therefore, the working hand will be the one that performs the thumb or finger walking and other techniques. Just remember: because each of the techniques mentioned here has its own special holding methods, you should not only be aware of the way the massages are done, but also how the foot is kept in place.

Holding the Foot
There are two types of holding: with the non-moving hand and by a reflex point using certain techniques. In the first type, the non-moving hand or holding hand (*one that keeps the foot down*) supports the foot being worked on, keeping it stable while providing the working hand with leverage. To hold the foot, place your thumb on the sole and your remaining fingers behind the foot. Most of the time, you may hold the foot near the ankle while you massage it with your moving hand.

On the other hand, holding on a reflex point may be used during certain techniques, especially while rotating, pressing or hooking and holding the foot. By rotating or pressing a certain point, the patient will experience a warm sensation throughout their body. This boosts the healing effect while clearing the pathway for energy to flow.

Stroking

Before you begin with the actual techniques of reflexology, you must warm up the foot. For this reason, the stroking method is ideal since it will help you stimulate the blood vessels of your patient's feet and promote gentle heat.

To begin with the stroking technique, hold the foot in your hands and start to massage the top of the foot gently. Remember to use your thumbs in a slow but firm stroking motion to avoid applying a lot of pressure initially. Stroking begins at the toes and you can move up to the ankle and finish the process by following the same line back to the toes. However, remember to apply slightly lighter pressure towards the ankles as this is a sensitive area.

Thumb Walking

Thumb walking is one of the best and most effective techniques that you can use for people facing kidney failure. While you are holding the foot, place the outside corner of your thumb on the top part of the leg. Bend the thumb a couple of times and do not worry about exerting too much pressure or inflicting pain. Next, push the thumb forward by walking it. Always use the outside tip of your thumb and bend it while rocking it a little to achieve the best results.

Finger Walking

The finger walking method is quite similar to the thumb walking technique. The only difference here is that you will be flexing the first joint of your finger instead of the thumb. If you are only starting out, you can use the top of your other hand as practice ground.

What you need to do is to hold the practice forearm or actual foot with two fingers and use another, preferably the index finger to walk with a slight rocking motion. Note that because of the leverage provided by the wrist and thumb of your hand, raising the wrists will increase the pressure while lowering them will decrease it. Also remember that when using this technique, you must move in the forward direction, never sideways or backwards, because this will defeat the entire purpose.

Pivoting

Another very good technique that you can use to help a person with kidney failure is pivoting. To practice this method, you should gently hold the foot in the holding hand and use the other to massage the sole of the foot with your thumb. To start the process, begin at the area directly below the large toe and work your way to below the rest of the toes. Once you have applied initial pressure, you can roll the thumb back and forth or wiggle it for a few second, release pressure and move on to the next area. This pivoting technique can be used for the ridges of the foot as well, which are related to the kidneys.

Wringing
The wringing technique is also called the ankle rotation method because it is focused on the ankle. For this method, you should first move the ankle side to side to gently loosen the joint. Next, use a cupping motion to hold the heel of the foot and use the holding hand to firmly hold the ball of the foot. Once the foot is in place, rotate the foot clockwise and anti clockwise three to four times so that the ankle joint is relaxed. You can change the pressure later but remember to not do so often or this will stress your patient.

Hook and Backup
The hook and backup technique is ideal if you need to apply pressure to a certain reflex point that is too deep or hard to reach or simply if you need to be precise. To start implementing the hook and backup, hold the foot with four fingers of the working hand. With your thumb, press firmly at the point.

During this technique, it is important that you keep the pressure steady and do not move the thumb from the reflex point. Instead, relax the tissues beneath by moving the thumb back and forth. However, be careful not to keep the thumb at one position for too long because this will strain and tense the muscles instead of relaxing them.

Zigzag Thumb Walk
Finally, among the top and most effective techniques, the zigzag thumb method comes highly recommended for patients with kidney failure. This technique is similar to thumb walking and resembles the movements that are made by shears when cutting a hem. To start the zigzag thumb walk, you should start at the base of the heel and use the right thumb to walk diagonally across the reflex points and then back to the point where you started. Remember that the thumb movement during this technique is slow, steady and very even.

The Butterfly Technique
The butterfly technique is a two-handed technique that allows reflexology practitioners to smooth out an area and work deeper on it. Both hands are used to hold the foot, with both thumbs on the sole and palms on top of it. To implement this technique, you need to move the thumbs towards the center of the foot and then back to the sole. Make sure that your thumbs look like butterfly wings while you're moving in and out.

Karate Chops
As tough as this reflexology technique may sound, this is one of the gentle and effective methods for kidney failure patients. It helps with circulation and usually signals the end of the session. To carry out this step, use quick chopping motions, especially around the heel ridge.

Clapping
This technique entails lightly slapping the entire foot area with an open hand. You need to clap the top, bottom and sides of the foot with either one or both hands. You can also alternate between using the palm of your hand and is back. However, while implementing this technique, you should use a steady, even pressure. In addition, you should be in tune with the treatment to feel any awkwardness while implementing it. That way, you can ensure your patient of the best and most relaxing treatment.

PARTING WORDS

Despite the great advances that modern medicine has been able to achieve, the problems kidney failure patients face cannot easily be solved. This is the reason why more and more people are starting to turn towards reflexology to relieve chronic pain, stress and other symptoms. The reflexology treatment is seen to be effective in innumerable health problems and issues and will help your loved one in more than one way.

Here are a few of the things you have learned while reading this entire booklet.

1. How reflexology works and the various studies conducted to prove its effectiveness with kidney failure patients
2. The zones that correspond to specific body parts such as the kidney
3. The various bones and areas which will benefit you when you start the reflexology sessions
4. The various considerations you must think of before starting with reflexology sessions.
5. The eight most commonly used techniques of reflexology and how to start practicing them on yourself and on the patient

Now that you have learned the basics of reflexology, you can bring relief to the ones you love simply by implementing its techniques mentioned in this chapters above. However, before you start with the sessions, consult with the patient's physician to find out about any complications that can reduce the effects of your reflexology treatment.

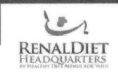

CRANIOSACRAL THERAPY
THE DO'S AND DON'TS TO FEEL RELIEF

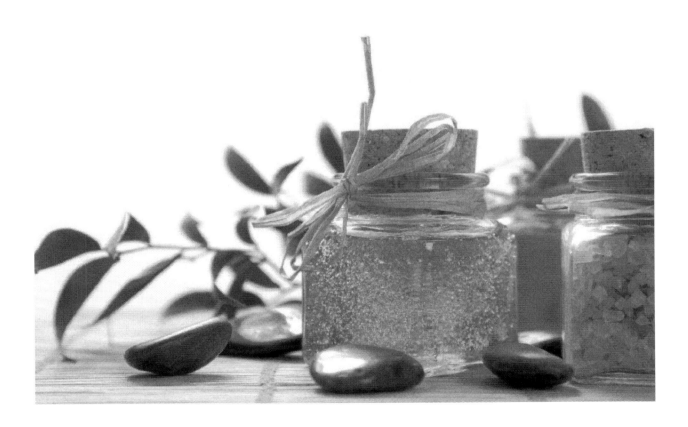

INTRODUCTION

For many patients suffering from chronic kidney disease, looking at alternative therapies for the relief of symptoms offers a more natural approach that they find less intrusive and gentler to their bodies. CranioSacral Therapy (CST) is a type of massage that is gaining in popularity for those suffering from chronic diseases since it can offer relief for a variety of symptoms and is non-invasive.

CranioSacral Therapy is a form of treatment that involves the therapist using a very light touch (about the weight of a nickel) to assist the release of any internal blockages or restrictions that might exist along the spinal column or within the cranium and sacrum. The objective of the therapy is to improve the operation of the central nervous system by balancing the flow of cerebrospinal fluid.

CranioSacral Therapy relies on normalizing the flow of cerebrospinal fluid by softly manipulating the bones, muscles, and connective tissue (fascia) through a relaxing massage process. For those with kidney failure, it could be beneficial for treating a variety of symptoms associated with chronic kidney disease including chronic pain, insomnia, hypertension, and depression.

The Cranial Rhythm

Dr. John Upledger, a graduate from Michigan State University, founded CranioSacral Therapy in the 1980s. It is an osteo therapy that is comparable to chiropractic therapy, only carried out with less pressure and less physical manipulation on the part of the therapist.

CranioSacral Therapy is based around adjusting the "Cranial Rhythm." The Cranial Rhythm, like breathing and the heartbeat, is a distinctive cadence inside the body- only this particular rhythm concerns the cerebrospinal fluid (CSF). In CranioSacral Therapy, it is thought that the rhythm can become imbalanced or that the fluid can become blocked and the central nervous system suffers. Consequently, this is believed to cause all sorts of problems within the body.

The central nervous system runs from your brain all the way down your spinal column. However, its functions aren't limited to these areas. The spinal cord gets information from the muscles, joints, connective tissue, and even the skin through nerve transmissions. Of course, the brain is a part of the central nervous system and also the most complicated. It gets information from your mouth and other fixtures on your face, but it uses your spinal cord to get information from the rest of your body. The nervous system is responsible for many functions within the body, including temperature control, your heartbeat when you're resting and when you're active, pain, and even blood pressure. Even your kidneys are affected. Part of the nervous system, for instance, contributes to arterial pressure control by modifying heart production and kidney function.

The Cerebral Spinal Fluid

The cerebrospinal fluid (CSF) is a clear liquid that surrounds the brain and spinal cord. Not only does it serve to protect the brain inside the skull, CSF also helps nutrients that have been filtered from the blood flow throughout the body and it eliminates certain toxins from the brain. Although the brain makes around 17 ounces of CSF every day, since the fluid is constantly being reabsorbed, there's only about 3-5 ounces present at any given moment.

The cerebrospinal fluid has four main functions. These are to provide:

1. **Buoyancy:** CSF allows the brain to keep its density without being brought down by its own weight, which is around 3 pounds. If it didn't have CSF

giving it buoyancy then its weight would cut off blood supply to the sections of the brain that didn't have any fluid available to them.

2. **Protection:** The cerebrospinal fluid protects the tissue of the brain from being damaged when the head is injured by offering a buffer of sorts.

3. **Waste management:** As the CSF flows through the inner ventricular system in the brain and is then absorbed back into the bloodstream, certain metabolic wastes are removed in the process. If this didn't happen and chemical disruptions occurred then it would be difficult to manage blood pressure and temperature.

4. **Avoidance of brain ischemia:** By constantly reabsorbing the CSF inside the skull as part of the hydraulic process, brain ischemia (a condition in which there is not enough blood flow to the brain, causing a type of stroke) is prevented. This also reduces the risk of complete intracranial pressure (swelling of the brain).

Although the cerebrospinal fluid is limited to the brain and spinal column, problems with it can affect the nervous system and issues with the nervous system can affect the entire body. CranioSacral Therapy targets the cerebrospinal fluid and helps that flow properly and functions correctly. When the cerebrospinal fluid can properly flow, the other systems in the body are able to function more competently.

The cerebrospinal fluid's pressure and volume fluctuate regularly, which makes it a hydraulic system. It needs to be constantly moving in order to transport nutrients to the neurons and to remove waste and toxins from the brain. CranioSacral Therapy facilitates the removal of any restrictions or blockages that might be causing the fluid to function improperly. As a result, the therapy can improve the health not only of the brain and spinal cord, but of the entire body.

How the Cranial Rhythm Works

The Cranial Rhythm, while similar to breathing and the heartbeat, is separate from these two rhythms. Is often described as the feeling of a "wave" or an impulse. Every therapist feels this in a different way. If an area is restricted or it feels blocked then the therapist might describe that particular area as feeling irregular or uneven.

Although the Cranial Rhythm involves the cerebrospinal fluid, any part of the body can be affected since the nervous system affects all bodily systems, from the digestive system to the skeletal system. During the therapy, the therapist will apply light pressure to the fascia (the connective tissue that surrounds the muscles, organs, bones, and nerves) and wait for the restrictions in that area to be released. Sometimes, a restriction on one part of the body can cause a problem in an entirely different location. For instance, the therapist might feel a restriction or imbalance in the Cranial Rhythm in your neck and this might be causing you to urinate less frequently. A restriction in your lower back may be causing pain in your head. CranioSacral Therapy believes that all systems are interconnected and dependent upon one another.

SOMATO EMOTIONAL RELEASE

In addition to the physical aspects of CranioSacral therapy, which includes releasing restrictions and blockages, a lot of therapists also believe that there is an emotional aspect to the CST treatment that is also beneficial to the patient as well.

Many practitioners believe that the body holds onto memories in our physical composition as well as in our minds. Most people are aware of the fact that they can have a physical response to a painful memory. When remembering something that causes them pain, they might find that their blood pressure momentarily increases, their heart rate increases, and they become tense and anxious. When the mind refuses to let go of any painful events and memories, these can become embedded into our physical makeup and cause restrictions within the body. These restrictions are sometimes referred to as an "energy cyst." Over time this can lead to very real physical symptoms such as chronic pain.

Treatment with CranioSacral Therapy can help therapists discover where those memories and correlating emotions are hidden and release them. As a result, the body can be released of any symptoms that might not have any medical reasons for existing.

The technique that is used to release these emotions is called Somato Emotional Release (SER). It focuses on a safe and efficient way of releasing painful emotions and memories so that they no longer cause any physical symptoms on the body. Through SER, the lingering effects of any distress that a patient may have suffered in the past can safely and effectively be released. The treatment allows the body to release any former trauma by relaxing and giving both the body and mind permission to "let go" of any negative thoughts and emotions that may have been lingering for far too long.

CranioSacral Therapy and Kidney Disease

CranioSacral Therapy may be very useful for those suffering from kidney failure, as it could provide relief from a variety of symptoms that are associated with chronic kidney disease. The therapy has been shown to reduce such symptoms as chronic pain, insomnia, and depression-all of which are known symptoms of chronic kidney disease. In addition, it has also been shown to help with high blood pressure, which is important for those experiencing kidney failure.

What conditions can CranioSacral Therapy address that might be valuable for CKD?

- Headaches
- Stress/anxiety
- Fatigue
- Urinary retention
- Hypertension
- Insomnia
- Chronic pain
- Fluid retention
- Depression

Stress and anxiety

Stress and anxiety are two common symptoms that those suffering from chronic kidney disease find themselves facing. Researchers found in a 2009 study published in "Evidence-Based Complementary and Alternative Medicine" that after 25 weeks of CranioSacral therapy patients experienced a substantial improvement not only in their level of pain but also in their anxiety and their overall quality of life.

Fatigue

Fatigue can be a symptom of chronic kidney disease and something that's challenging to deal with since it can be difficult to perform the activities that most patients enjoy doing. It can even interfere with job and parenting duties. However, many patients claim that after having just one session with CranioSacral Therapy they walk away feeling rejuvenated and relaxed. After having a few sessions, they begin feeling an increased sense of vitality and wellbeing. With improved sleep and less pain, this can oftentimes improve energy levels as well.

Urinary Retention

Sometimes, if there is an energy cyst or restriction near an organ, it can cause problems with that organ. This is commonly seen in issues with the bowels and kidneys. Naturally, where chronic kidney disease is concerned, it's important to flush out toxins and encourage urination-although some dialysis diets limit the amount of fluids that you're allowed to drink. Being able to empty the bladder is especially important to patients with chronic kidney disease because a backup of urine can send toxins back into the kidneys.

By correcting the cerebrospinal fluid flow and bringing the Cranial Rhythm back into balance, some patients find that they no longer suffer from the urinary retention that they suffered from in the past. They are able to start urination, urinate more frequently and empty their bladders completely. If there was a restriction close to their bladder or kidneys and this is released then this can also be helpful in stimulating the urination process for the patient.

High Blood Pressure

There are several ways in which CranioSacral Therapy can help lessen hypertension. When the brain and central nervous system use nutrients from the increased blood flow and cerebrospinal fluid, the brain chemistry stabilizes and the body's emotions can alter in a positive way. When the therapist works with the spine, sacrum, and cranium through CST, the therapy techniques basically retune the nervous system by bringing the Cranial Rhythm to a momentary standstill. This standstill is a positive thing since it allows the nervous system to relax for a moment and make any corrections it needs to. It's effectively "resetting." This is sometimes called a "parasympathetic shift." Stress, anxiety, and tension can be moved into a more balanced state during this time as the mind moves from a fight or flight response. With ongoing treatment sessions, a lot of patients have seen a reduction of high blood pressure associated with CranioSacral Therapy. This might be due to the therapy's influence on the nervous system and the relaxation that it provides for both the mind and the body.

Insomnia

Sometimes, structural restrictions can affect the autonomic nervous system. The autonomic nervous system regulates the functions of the internal organs sort of like an automated system or program. The parasympathetic nervous system is one of three branches of the autonomic nervous system and is responsible for relaxing and renewing your body after it's been exposed to stress or activity. It essentially helps you rest and rejuvenates you while you sleep. It slows down your heart rate, stimulates digestion, stores energy, and dilates the blood vessels.

CranioSacral Therapy can encourage the parasympathetic nervous system to work at its optimal performance. Boosting the parasympathetic system's performance can improve the body's capacity to rest and heal. With therapy, some benefits have included increased REM sleep which means decreased insomnia, too. In one study reported to the *Journal of Hypertension* in 2002 (20:2063-2068) it was discovered that CranioSacral therapy reduced the time it took for patients to fall asleep. It accomplished this by reducing the sympathetic tone of the nervous system (the other branch of the autonomic nervous system).

Chronic pain

CranioSacral Therapy has been successfully used to identify the source of pain and release the patterns that are causing it. This has been especially beneficial as far as lower back pain and headaches are concerned. In CST it is thought that pain could be the result of decreased blood flow to an area, an accumulation of metabolic waste products, a pressure on the nervous system tissues, and even just a general sense of fatigue.

In chronic kidney disease, nerve strain caused by a muscular imbalance, tension, or infection might cause excessive sensitivity of local nociceptors (nerve cell endings that start the awareness of pain). This can make it feel as though there is a continuous reverberation of pain being sent to the brain. By releasing any restrictions and lightly massaging areas close to the joints and spine to relax the muscles, the signals of pain will no longer be sent to the brain at such a fast pace. This can be helpful for several types of pain, including lower back pain and headaches.

Fluid retention

One of the benefits of CranioSacral Therapy is that it can boost fluid movement through the body. If the therapy is carried out regularly, it can help reduce fluid retention and swelling since it helps release the fluid in the body instead of gathering in one place.

Depression

Some patients with chronic kidney disease suffer from depression, especially if they feel as though they are limited from enjoying activities or foods they used to take pleasure from. CranioSacral Therapy has been used to treat depression in a couple of different ways. Sometimes, by merely ensuring the cerebrospinal fluid is mobile and freely flowing throughout the body and the rhythm is back in balance again it's enough to counteract the symptoms of depression.

If the depression lingers, then a triad compression might be present in the base of the skull. A triad compression is three areas of tightness in the upper and lower spine and in the head. By releasing these compressions using the CranioSacral Therapy techniques, not only could the symptoms of depression be lessened (or disappear) but other symptoms associated with the compression might also be targeted as well. Those symptoms include lower back pain, headaches, and sciatica.

The Treatment Process

The specific treatment process will vary a little bit depending on the center and the therapist, but for the most part it will work the same way. There is both a physical and an emotional aspect to being treated and therefore it's important that the patient feels rapport and trust with the therapist. In order for the therapy to work, the therapist must be mindful of the patient's needs and stop if they find that the patient is becoming uncomfortable, especially in regards to SER (somato emotional release).

How the treatment process works

First, patients will give the therapist their medical history and talk about any problems they are having. They also discuss what they hope to accomplish during the sessions. As with any doctor's appointment, the patient and therapist will talk about any preexisting conditions or medical problems that the patient has. (It's important to keep in mind, however, that the CST therapist is not a replacement for your doctor, the questions will help them determine where to start looking for restrictions and blockages.)

During the treatment process, the patient is fully clothed and lies on a massage table. Depending on which technique the therapist is using, the patient might lie on their back, side, or stomach. It's a full body treatment. A massage therapist places his or her hands on different parts of the client's body, usually starting with the head. They search for areas where the Cranial Rhythm might be "off" and lightly massage the muscles, bones, and connective tissues of those areas.

To release the blockages, the therapist lightly manipulates the tissues that surround the brain and spinal cord. Because the tissues can't be reached directly, the therapist lightly manipulates the bones with a gentle touch in order to access the membranes and tissues. During the treatment, the therapist may move different parts of the body including the arms and legs and feel the spine, ribcage and cranium. They are doing this as they search for areas that might have limited flow.

How often treatment is needed

The number of sessions generally depends on the patient and how often they feel like they need it. In most cases, patients need about 5 treatments with a gap of 1-2 weeks between the first few. Some patients require them more frequently, which is why family members might learn how to give them at home.

With someone who has chronic kidney disease, maintenance treatments might be needed to help manage insomnia, hypertension, and pain. This is something the patient can talk about with the therapist. A maintenance visit would not typically last as long as a regular session.

What does it feel like?
Once the treatment is over, is there any pain?

The touch that is used during the treatment is very light. It's been compared to the pressure of lightly touching a coin to the skin. There isn't any pain involved, although some patients do feel as though their tissue is being slightly stretched. This isn't described as an uncomfortable or painful sensation.

Some patients end up feeling a little lightheaded and some have slight headaches for a day or two. Others claim to feel better almost immediately. The benefits of the therapy are meant to be cumulative, with the best results felt after several treatments.

During the session, some patients:

- Feel so relaxed that they want to fall asleep.
- Enter a meditative state.
- Feel as though they're both dreaming and awake at the same time.
- Experience memories they had forgotten about.
- Feel as though they're floating above the table.

When the session is over, many patients find that they:

- Have a lot of energy.
- Are able to breathe more deeply.
- Have better posture.
- Feel a sense of renewal and peace.
- Sleep well; with less trouble falling asleep and have the ability to stay asleep.

After the treatment, the patient might feel some other sensations as well. If they have been constipated, for instance, then they might find that the bowels are "gurgling" and there is a need to use the restroom. There might also be the need to urinate. Most people, however, feel very relaxed and rejuvenated.

Precautions

In one study, 5% of those with preexisting head injuries felt worse after treatment. As a result, CST treatment is not recommended if you have had a recent head trauma or skull fracture, have a disease that affects the brain or spinal cord, or suffer from a condition in which a change in CSF pressure might be dangerous to the brain.

Because it can create such a relaxing experience and cause drowsiness and light-headedness, it is usually advised that patients avoid driving or operating any heavy machinery immediately following CranioSacral Therapy.

CranioSacral Therapists

A therapist trained to perform CranioSacral Therapy should be certified, although there is no standard licensing board for these kinds of therapists. The practitioners who are trained in CST can range from massage therapists to physical therapists who have specialized training in the field. In addition, family members and friends can also learn the techniques so that patients can continue to receive treatment and relief at home.

When it comes to being certified, some states do not have any requirements for those who offer massages like CranioSacral Therapy (CST) or MyoFascial Release (MFR) while others do.

Certification programs

Therapists can go through certification programs and train to become CranioSacral therapists. These are nationally certified professionals. These professionals might only be CranioSacral therapists and only practice this kind of therapy, although they might also do other types of bodywork.

During the certification programs, the therapists are trained to find the areas on the patient's body where their energy might be blocked or there are restrictions in the muscles or fascia (the structure of connective tissue that surrounds the muscles, groups of muscles, blood vessels, and nerves) that must be released. The therapists are specially trained to find and correct the imbalances within the body by helping the cerebrospinal fluid properly flow.

The Biodynamic CranioSacral Therapy Association of North America (https://www.craniosacraltherapy.org/) is one non-profit organization that supports practitioners and schools of the biodynamic model of Craniosacral therapy. It employs a curriculum for training and provides a referral service for Registered CranioSacral therapists. The Upledger Institute (www.upledger.com/) also offers a CranioSacral Therapy certification program and offers a database to help clients find practitioners. In addition, the Upledger Institute offers the American CranioSacral Therapy Association that practitioners can belong to which helps ensure quality and performance by therapists.

Abroad, the CranioSacral Therapy Association (http://www.craniosacral.co.uk/) located in the United Kingdom has a practitioner directory and links to training sites. The International Affiliation of Biodynamic Trainings (http://biodynamic-craniosacral.org/) has several schools around the world under its affiliation and provides high standards, a professional code of conduct, and more than 1,000 practitioners in its database.

Since there can be different levels of certification, you can always ask about your therapist's background and specialty. In addition, to feel more comfortable, you can also ask which level they studied and how often they perform CST.

Massage therapists & other healers

A lot of healers who practice CranioSacral Therapy have diverse backgrounds which include osteopathy, massage, shiatsu, and acupuncture. Massage therapists, particularly, often add CST to their treatment list since it is so closely related to massage.

In some cases, a massage therapist may have a certification in CranioSacral Therapy. Although a CST might not have to be certified to practice, a massage therapist in the United States must be licensed to practice massage. The body responsible for this is the National Certification Board for Therapeutic Massage and Body Work (http://www.ncbtmb.org/). It is illegal in all states to practice massage professionally without a license.

When a massage therapist also practices CranioSacral Therapy, they have probably undergone additional training for this. There are various programs located throughout the country that offer this certification so if you are considering getting work done by a massage therapist you might first ask if they are licensed and then ask where they received their training for the CST. You can also ask if they belong to any CranioSacral organizations or associations and have any professional affiliations.

Family and loved ones

It is also possible for family members to take classes (usually only lasting a couple of hours) to learn how to do the techniques at home so that they can continue the therapy with their loved ones in order to offer relief on a more frequent basis. These classes can be offered at healing arts academies or other institutions that offer trainings in complementary or alternative health therapies. Your therapist can usually give this information to you during your appointment if you are interested in learning more information. Keep in mind, however, that not every institution offers this service and that charges usually apply. Sometimes, these charges will be minimal, especially if you are a family member of a patient. Other times, you might be required to become completely certified. If this happens, you might expect to pay as much as $300-500.

SIMPLE TECHNIQUES TO TRY AT HOME

For the caregiver, there are some simple techniques that can be used with CranioSacral Therapy with the patient at home, even without professional training.

Tip: Remember, when performing the therapy, the patient must be comfortable. Although most patients will position themselves on a table, others find this uncomfortable and some prefer to sit in a chair (this limits the body parts you're able to access, of course). The pressure that should be applied to the body is about that of what you would use to press a coin into the skin. Be gentle and soothing. This is not a typical kind of massage, where you are kneading the muscles or trying to manipulate any muscles or joints. This requires a light touch.

EXERCISE ONE: FASCIAL UNWINDING

Fascial unwinding allows the body to release stress and any other weaknesses that are holding it back from performing at its optimal level. The fascia is connective tissue that runs throughout the body. It surrounds the bones and connecting muscles and, through its currents, transmits signals to the rest of your body at a quick speed.

To begin with, you must try to figure out where on the patient's body they are experiencing any fascial restriction. Fascial restrictions can be found all over the body, but tend to be more common along the spine. You can search for them by gently resting your hands on different parts of the patient's body and attempting to identify any tension within the fascia. This takes concentration on the part of you, the practitioner, and most people find that going into a slight meditative state is helpful.

The pulls and tension will probably be subtle. When they are located, however, try to visualize lines extending from those points and all gathering into one certain focal point in the body. This is referred to as the "source of restriction." If it helps, visualize that source on the body as magnet, with lines from the tension-filled areas being drawn to it.

Next, you'll place both of your hands on that part of the body and apply light pressure over it. Lightly manipulate the tissue by slightly pushing on it. You are essentially envisioning it "releasing" or dissolving. The goal is to get fascial release, or unwinding, to occur so that the tissues will become more balanced. As a result, they will no longer be out of alignment and the patient won't feel tension or any pulls in that area. As a result, the lines extending from that point will also dissolve.

This exercise can be performed on any body part, including the trunk, stomach, or leg. It can also be used to help facilitate the breaking up of adhesions in old scar tissue from previous surgeries. For chronic kidney disease, if the patient is experiencing any lower back pain then this is something that you might want to consider trying on the trunk or lower back for pain relief. Although the tension is released from the one focal area, most patients experience a generalized release of tension, too, and come away feeling relaxed all over.

EXERCISE TWO: CRANIAL BASE RELEASE

The Cranial Base Release concentrates on a trapped **occipital-atlantal joint**, which is located at the base of the skull and is the first joint in the neck. When it becomes trapped, or fixated, it can cause headaches, insomnia, and even vertigo. For the patient with chronic kidney disease, working with CST on this area may help improve sleep and headaches.

To begin with, the patient lies flat on their back on the table. The practitioner then places both of their hands in a cupped position and rests the patients head and neck on their fingertips. If positioned correctly, the finger tips should be at the base of the patient's skull under their Occipital Ridge (the area at the back of the head where the skull meets the spine).

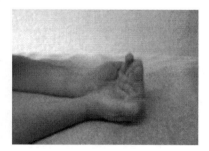

From here on, all you need are gravity and the patient's own head for the exercise to work. The weight of head helps open up the channels for energy flow and as the balance starts to occur again, the back of the patient's head will drop back into the practitioner's hands. Their chin should then rise up.

Exercise Three: Sphenoid Adjustment

The third exercise involves the sphenoid. A small bone behind the eyes, the liquid motion of the cerebral spinal fluid eventually causes the sphenoid to slightly shift. Sometimes, it can move a great deal. Most of the time, the movement of the sphenoid jolts the pituitary gland. If the sphenoid is moving improperly, then this can have an effect on endocrine system function since the pituitary gland overseas many of the body's systems.

To begin the exercise, have your patient lie down on a table. Place your hands on either side of their head and let your thumbs rest on their temple. Your pinky should be able to reach the occiput (the lower back portion of the head), but if it isn't then just let your fingers rest where they can.

As the cerebrospinal fluid is made, the sphenoid should move downward since the cranial vault expands. As the fluid is absorbed, the sphenoid should move upward. Visualizing the movement of the cerebrospinal fluid, lightly move your hands up and down, using slight pressure, and feeling the sphenoid under your fingertips.

You will probably notice that the motion of the sphenoid is slightly off balance. As you find the rhythm of the cerebrospinal fluid, however, and are able to visualize it, you should notice that as it moves back to the joint with the occiput it eventually becomes freer and more relaxed. This is because tension is being released.

Continue doing this for several minutes, or a few cycles of fluid, until the tension has been released.

Exercise Four: The Pelvic Release

There is a great amount of energy flow through the pelvic region for both men and women. Not only are there emotions associated with it that the body can remember, but the pelvic area can also be a source of pain, too, as it can hold scar tissue, bladder issues, and memories of child birth. For those with chronic kidney disease, the pelvic region is especially important to focus on.

This release is meant to help let go of any tension and pressure and to help with any chronic pain in this area. It is also a relaxing exercise that might be valuable to those with hypertension.

To start, sit next to your client in a chair. Using the hand closest to them, place it on their lower back until it touches their sacrum. Using your other hand, rest it on their lower abdomen. Move it downwards until the edge of your hand touches the top of their pubic bone. Do not apply a lot of pressure; use only a slight, gentle touch.

Lightly, move your hand back up the abdomen and stop until it rests mid-stomach. Then, slowly move it back down until it touches the top of the pubic bone again. Repeat this several times, while keeping your other hand on their sacrum. Try to listen and feel for the rhythm of their body and cerebrospinal fluid and visual the pressure and tension being released from their pelvis region.

EXERCISE FIVE: RANGE OF MOTION

In this exercise, you're focusing on the neck and the spinal column.

You start out by having the patient lie on their back with their head resting comfortably on a table, or on the bed. Standing behind them, gentle lift their head and cradle it in your hands so that their neck is supported. Gently move their head from side to side, turning their head to face first one side and then the other. Also move their head up and down several times. This is to ensure that their neck has proper range of motion. If this becomes uncomfortable for the patient, then stop.

Once the neck is warmed up, gently press down on both shoulders several times to help relax those muscles.

Next, place both hands under the neck at the base and gently bring your fingers up the skin to the hairline in a "wave" motion. Do this several times in order to help stimulate the Cranial Rhythm.

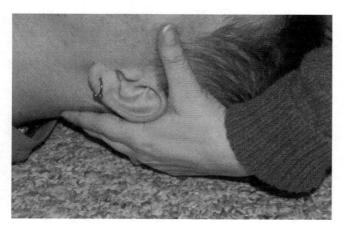

You can then perform a Cranial Base Release if the patient has been experiencing any headaches or neck pain. This will be an added bonus, especially since you are already working with the neck and cranium.

Finish by lightly pressing into the Occipital Ridge (the space at the back of the head where the lower part of the skull meets the spine) several times with your knuckles and then making the "wave" motion" from the base of the neck up to the hairline at least four times before stopping.

EXERCISE SIX: LOWER BACK RELEASE
This is a good technique for those patients who are suffering from lower back pain or any disturbances in the lower quadrant.

The patient will lie on their stomach on a table for this treatment. They can be fully clothed if they feel more comfortable that way. Start by lightly massaging the sacrum (the triangle shaped area where the lower back meets the pelvis) and pushing downwards from the spinal column, searching for any tension in the lower back. If you feel any compression, rather than pushing on it or "kneading" it, lightly touch it, shift it, and manipulate it in a circular motion.

When you feel the tension soften, move your hand away and lightly massage the area around the restriction. You will probably find that this area is now noticeably softer as well.

Lastly, place one hand at the top of the spine and the other hand on the sacrum and apply gentle pressure to both places. Let your hands rest here for a few seconds, feeling the Cranial Rhythm.

CONCLUSION

It's always important to talk to your doctor before embarking on any other therapies in regards to your kidney disease. Although CranioSacral Therapy is considered safe, and there are no known harmful side effects for the majority of patients, it's important to be on the same page with your medical team and inform them of any other therapies you might be undertaking.

For those suffering from kidney failure, CST should be considered a complementary therapy to any other therapy that is recommended by a physician and is generally not expected to be a standalone treatment. It shouldn't be dependent upon as the singular treatment for kidney failure. Still, many patients claim that after receiving several treatments they notice a significant increase in their overall wellness and vitality, as well as a reduction in their chronic pain and any emotional disturbances they may have been afflicted with. CranioSacral Therapy's benefits might not be noticeable right away, but it can help the body rejuvenate all of its systems so that it learns to heal itself more effectively. As a result, some patients continue to notice improvements for weeks after their session has ended.

WORKSHEETS SECTION

You have copies of the worksheets in the following pages, and the individual files are available when you sign up at this link: **www.renaldiethq.com/caregiverworksheets**. This allows us to send you updated copies if things change or errors are noted. To print the files from the email you will need adobe acrobat.

Worksheets Included

1. Initial Visit to MD Worksheet
2. Follow Up Doctor Visit Worksheet
3. Medication Worksheet
4. Allergies and Conditions Worksheet
5. Questions for the Doctor
6. Personal Condition Overview
7. Sleep Log
8. Exercise Log
9. Healthy Eating for CKD Worksheets
10. Treatment for Low Blood Sugar
11. Managing Fluid Intake

Initial Visit To Doctor Worksheet

Name: _____ Date Completed: _____

Please indicate issues within each area for your medical history (items listed are some potential issues but not all inclusive):

1. General: (Fever, Chills, Overall Health)
   _____
   _____
   _____

2. Eyes (vision problems, blurred vision, loss of vision, surgeries, eye pain)
   _____
   _____
   _____

3. Ears/Mouth/Throat (Dizziness, Dental Problems, Swollen glands in neck, Sore throat/pain when swallowing/ mouth sores)
   _____
   _____
   _____

4. Cardiovascular (chest pain, heart racing, shortness of breath, leg pain in calf or thigh, fainting spells, swelling of legs)
   _____
   _____
   _____

5. Breathing/Respiratory (Shortness of breath, night sweats, coughing up blood, chronic cough, hayfever, seasonal allergies)
   _____
   _____
   _____

6. Gastrointestinal (decreased appetite, nausea/vomiting, constipation, increased appetite, stomach pain, diarrhea)
   _____
   _____
   _____

Initial Visit To Doctor Worksheet

Name: _____ Date Completed: _____

7. Genitourinary (Men and Women—pain when urinating, urinating more than normal, pain during sex, sores (vagina, penis, rectum), blood in urine, bladder infection, changes in sex drive) (Women—irregular periods, increased or decreased bleeding during menstruation, yeast infections, painful periods, discharge or unusual smell from vagina) (Men—discharge from penis (drip), swelling in balls (scrotum))

_____
_____
_____

8. Musculoskeletal (joint pain, numbness/tingling/weakness in arms or legs, limited motion of arms/legs, swelling or redness, pain in calf or thigh))

_____
_____
_____

9. Neurological (nervous system issues, arm/leg weakness, new headaches, headaches with vision changes, repeated bad headaches, migraines, problems with memory/speech)

_____
_____
_____

10. Psychiatric (suicidal thoughts, seeing or hearing things (hallucinations), mood swings)

_____
_____
_____

11. Endocrine (thirsty all the time, increased facial hair (women), weight gain/loss, cannot stand temperature changes (hot or cold), kidney problems, stage of kidney failure)

_____
_____
_____

Initial Visit To Doctor Worksheet

Name: _____ Date Completed: _____

12. Lymph (swollen glands in armpits or groin)
_____
_____

13. Skin (changes in skin (bumps, moles, tone), rash (palms of hands, soles of feet), sores or rash on skin)
_____
_____
_____

14. Allergies (hives or skin rashes, allergic reaction to drugs, allergic reaction to foods)
_____
_____
_____

15. Other conditions or issues
_____
_____
_____
_____
_____
_____

Follow Up Visit To Doctor Worksheet

Name: _____ Date Completed: _____

1. What is your main concern? _____

2. Do you have any new symptoms, or pains, that you have noticed since the last visit?
   _____
   _____

3. What changes have you noticed in your health since your last visit?
   _____
   _____

4. How do you feel your medications are working for control of your symptoms or disease? Are they still effective or do they seem to have decreased effects?
   _____
   _____

5. Have you started any new medications? (Both over the counter, herbal, or from other doctors) What are they and what dose are you taking? Have you noticed any side effects or changes?
   _____
   _____

6. Have you seen other doctors between our visits? If so, what for and what are the results? Have you had any tests done we should talk about?
   _____
   _____

Follow Up Visit To Doctor Worksheet

Name: _____ Date Completed: _____

Notes from this visit:

1. Tests ordered

   _____
   _____

2. Test results

   _____
   _____

3. Recommendations from Doctor

   _____
   _____

4. Medication Instructions

   _____
   _____

5. Dietary restrictions or changes

   _____
   _____

6. Next steps or how long until follow up

   _____
   _____

7. Other notes:

Medication Tracking Worksheet

Name: _____ Date Completed: _____ Ht: _____ Wt: _____

- Use a pencil so changes can be made
- Do not list medications you will be taking for less than 2 weeks (antibiotics, etc)
- List all medications you are taking, incl. prescriptions, eye drops, inhalers/nebulizers, oxygen, creams and ointments, over the counter meds, etc

Name of Medication	Reason for Use	Description of Pill and Form	Dose taken	How much you take and when?	Prescribed by Doctor or Over the counter?	Start Date	Any special instructions?
Example: Ibuprofen	Chronic knee pain	Round, orange pill tablet	200 mg	Take 2 tablets in the morning with breakfast	Dr. Who	1/1/2014	Make sure to take with food

RENAL DIET HEADQUARTERS

Medication Tracking Worksheet

Name: _____ Date Completed: _____ Ht: _____ Wt: _____

Name of Medication	Reason for Use	Description of Pill and Form	Dose taken	How much you take and when?	Prescribed by Doctor or Over the counter?	Start Date	Any special instructions?

Allergies and Conditions Worksheet

Name: _____   Date Completed: _____

- Use a pencil so changes can be made
- List known allergies, diagnoses, and related conditions.

Allergy or Condition	Signs and Symptoms	Medication used to control	Emergency treatments	Doctor Name/ Number for condition

Allergies and Conditions Worksheet

Name: _____ Date Completed: _____

Allergy or Condition	Signs and Symptoms	Medication used to control	Emergency treatments	Doctor Name/ Number for condition

Questions to Ask The Doctor

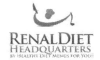

If starting a new medication—ask:

> What is the name of the medication and what is it supposed to do?
> Why is this the right medication for my condition, age, and gender?
> Are there things besides medications that help my condition or symptoms?
> If yes, how do these medications compare in safety, effectiveness, and price?
> What results will I get from this and how long will that take?
> What are the side effects?
> Will this medication work safely with ALL my other medications?
> How do I take this medication? When do I start and stop?
> What should I do if I forget or miss a dose?
> Should I avoid certain foods, alcohol, dietary supplements, over the counter medications, or driving while taking this medication?

If you need to see another doctor for a condition—ask:

> When will I be contacted by the other doctor/provider for an appointment?
> What should I expect them to do for my condition?
> Do I need any labs or other procedures to help them make their decisions about treatment?

If you are concerned about a condition the patient has and you feel has not been addressed—ask:

> How serious is the condition and how will it affect my work/life?
> What symptoms should I watch for?
> Is there more than one disease or condition that could be causing problems?
> Will I need more medical tests?
> Do I need a follow up visit and if so, when?
> If my symptoms worsen, what should I do on my own? When should I contact you?

If you need surgery and have questions—ask:

> Why do I need surgery?
> What surgical procedure are you recommending?
> Is there more than one way of performing this surgery?
> Are there alternatives to surgery?
> How much will surgery cost?
> What are the benefits of having surgery?
> What are the risks of having surgery?
> What if I don't have this surgery?
> Where can I get a second opinion?
> What kind of anesthesia will I need?
> How long will it take me to recover?
> What are your qualifications?
> How much experience do you have performing this surgery?
> How long will I be in the hospital?

Personal Condition/Information Overview

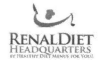

My Personal Information

Name: _____

Date of Birth: _____

Phone Number: _____

Allergies: (food or drug) _____

Emergency Contact Information

Name: _____

Relationship: _____

Phone Number: _____

Address: _____

Primary Care Physician

Name: _____

Phone Number: _____

Address: _____

Pharmacy/ Drugstore Information

Name: _____ Phone Number: _____

Address: _____

Other Physicians I See

Name: _____

Specialty: _____

Phone Number: _____

Name: _____

Specialty: _____

Phone Number: _____

Name: _____

Specialty: _____

Phone Number: _____

My Medical Conditions

_____

_____

_____

_____

_____

_____

_____

_____

_____

Name: _____

Sleep / Rest Log

Dates Completed: _____

Date	Time Sleeping	Hours Slept	Describe sleep—restful, tossing/turning, unable to sleep, etc.	How did you feel that day? Anything happen that affected sleep?
Example: 1/1/2014	9 pm—5 am	8 hours overnight	Restless, woke up many times	Tired, stress at work, woke up thinking about what I need to do at work

RENALDIET HEADQUARTERS

Exercise Tracking Log

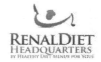

Name: _____   Dates Completed: _____

Date	Activity Done	Time	Notes/Comments about exercise
Example: 1/1/2014	Chair DVD	30 minutes	Difficult, had to stop many times but made it all 30 minutes

Healthy Eating For Chronic Kidney Disease

Why What You Eat Matters For CKD

Kidneys are a very important part of the way your body removes waste products from your blood. These add up and affect the way you feel. A special diet can help control the buildup of waste products and improve how you feel.

Pay attention to the following types of foods and minerals in your diet:

- **Protein**—before dialysis starts, you need to follow a lower protein diet to limit the build up of waste in your blood stream. After you start dialysis, you eat a higher amount of protein to replace what you lose during dialysis. Protein sources include beef, poultry, fresh pork, fish, seafood, and eggs.

- **Carbohydrates**—over half of the people diagnosed with chronic kidney disease have diabetes. You should continue to watch your carbohydrate count and monitor your blood sugar. This will help your body to stay balanced. Carbohydrate sources include breads, pastas, fruit, juices, starchy vegetables, and milks.

- **Sodium (salt)** - when your kidneys are not working at their optimum, they have a hard time removing salt from your bloodstream. Too much sodium can raise your blood pressure, increase your thirst, and cause swelling in your arms and legs. This adds strain to your heart and lungs. Avoid salting food at the table, using canned foods, eating fast foods, eating canned soups, and using salty seasonings such as garlic salt.

- **Potassium**—this mineral is found in many foods and keeps your muscles and heart working properly. Too much or too little can cause problems that are life threatening. You may need to limit high-potassium foods like potatoes, tomatoes and tomato products, melons, oranges, dairy products, and bananas. Avoid salt substitutes that contain potassium chloride as well.

- **Phosphorus**—this is another mineral that is found in almost all foods. You may have to limit this if you have too high levels in your blood. When it's too high, it pulls calcium out of your bones and make them brittle and weak. Dairy products are high in phosphorus, but other foods you may need to limit are: whole grain foods, dried beans and peas, nuts, peanut butter, and regular colas. You may take phosphate binders, and if you do you should take them with meals.

- **Calcium**—may need to be regulated. Calcium is usually highly regulated by your body, so ask your doctor if you have questions about your blood levels.

- **Fluids**—You might have additional fluid that your body cannot remove because of your condition. This fluid builds up in your hands, feet, lungs and heart and may make it harder to breathe and walk. Fluid restrictions are provided by your doctor.

Healthy Eating For Chronic Kidney Disease

Meal Planning Tips

Try to eat 3 meals each day—no less. Eating one or two large meals a day may cause weight gain.

Avoid delaying or skipping meals—Spacing meals evenly throughout the day will help you to avoid overeating.

If you tend to get hungry late at night, either plan a bedtime snack, or go to bed earlier to resist the temptation to eat.

Keep foods only in the kitchen, out of sight. Avoid putting dishes filled with candy, nuts, or other snacks in other rooms in the house.

Try to dine out only 2-3 times per week. Researchers have found that those dining out more often gain weight more easily.

Grocery Shopping Tips

Never go to the grocery store when hungry. Always try to eat your scheduled meal or snack before heading to the store.

Always have a grocery list ready and avoid buying foods not on your list. You will not only stick to your diet better, but also spend less money!

Choose more fresh foods like meat, produce, and dairy products. Foods that are ready to eat such as lunch meats, casseroles, desserts, and snack items often have the most fat and calories.

Try to grocery shop once a week instead of more often. That way you are more likely to stick to your list and plan your meals ahead.

Preparing Meals

Cut down on fat calories

- Use a non stick oil spray instead of frying oil in a pan
- Try using crumb mixtures and baking meat in the oven instead of deep fat frying.
- Trim the fat from meats, remove the skin from poultry, and drain the grease from hamburger.
- Use herbs, spices, and imitation butter flavoring to season foods.
- Use skim milk or non fat dry milk for recipes that call for milk
- Use fat free or reduced fat dairy products

Healthy Eating For Chronic Kidney Disease

Preparing Meals

Cut down on Empty Calories

- Instead of sugar, use sugar substitute in recipes and to sweeten foods. Many new sugar substitutes can be used measure for measure and cooked at a high temperature.
- Avoid alcohol. Alcohol such as wine, beer, and other liquors contain extra calories that are more easily stored as fat in the body.

Eating Meals

Eat Slowly—The brain needs about 20 minutes for the body to register that I has had enough food.

Take small bites and chew them well. Savor and enjoy every bite of food. This will help you eat slowly.

Always sit down to eat, and eat only in one place, preferably at the kitchen table.

Serve meals from the kitchen, not family style at the table.

Tips for Eating Out On A Renal Diet

Overall hints:

- Always remember your nutrition plan limits
- Plan meals in advance so it fits your nutrition needs (look on website for restaurant if possible)
- Consume only the fluids allowed for the event/meal; remember your fluid limit
- Practice good portion control with meals
- Share a meal with a friend
- Request low sodium options

Breakfast:

- Choose fried, poached or scrambled eggs
- Avoid high salt breakfast meat like bacon and sausage
- Select white toast, an English muffin or a bagel
- Skip bran or whole wheat muffins or bread
- Request cream cheese instead of cheddar or American cheese in an omelet
- Choose canned fruit as a side item instead of home fries or hash browns

Healthy Eating For Chronic Kidney Disease

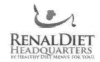

Beverages:

- Choose water, coffee, tea, non cola soda, cranberry, apple, or grape juice
- Skip colas and beer

Lunch and Dinner:

- Request low sodium broth based soups
- Choose beef, chicken, or fish tacos with lettuce and sour cream
- Select coleslaw or a green salad with chicken or shrimp
- Try low potassium vegetables on sandwiches to add lots of taste and flavor
- Limit extra meat and cheese on cold sandwiches and add vegetables instead
- Stick to white rice with natural seasoning instead of potatoes for side dishes
- Choose white pasta with herbs, olive oil, and garlic flavoring
- Order entrees prepared grilled, poached or roasted
- Try Angel food cake with strawberries, sherbet, or sorbet for dessert
- Skip soups unless they are low sodium
- Skip chocolate and carrot cake desserts

For Those With Diabetes and Renal Disease: Carbohydrates and Meal Planning

This table gives an approximate number of carbohydrate choices that should be eaten at each meal based on the calorie level you need each day. The amount you eat of carbohydrates helps control blood sugar levels, and must be combined with the recommended amount of protein and fat in the diet.

15 grams of carbohydrate = 1 carbohydrate choice

	1200 calories	1500 calories	1800 calories	2000 calories	2200 calories
Breakfast Carb Choices	3	3	4	4	5
Lunch Carb Choices	3	4	5	5	6
Dinner Carb Choices	3	5	4	6	6
Snack Carb Choices	1	1	1	1	1
Approximate total carb (45—55% of total calories)	135—165	170—205	200—245	225—275	250—300

Healthy Eating For Chronic Kidney Disease

Estimating The Size Of Protein Servings

Choose foods high in protein by using the following tips:

1. Chicken, turkey, fish, lean red meats, and egg whites are good sources of protein.
2. Dairy products such as milk, cheese, and yogurt also contain protein, but they can be high in fat, cholesterol, and phosphorus.
3. Meats that are "pink" such as: ham, bologna, hot dogs, sausage, salami, and any processed or canned meat are high in sodium and should be limited.

To estimate the portion size of Protein—use the following rules of thumb:

3 ounce serving of chicken or beef—deck of playing cards

3 ounce serving of fish—checkbook

1 slice of lunchmeat—Compact disc

1 medium egg—1 ounce of meat

1/4 cup egg substitute—1 golf ball—1 egg

Remember to remove the chicken skin to reduce the fat. You can do this after cooking. Bake, broil, roast, grill or boil meats for the lowest fat. If your foods are getting dry, use some non-stick cooking spray to moisten the meat. Trim off the fat before cooking. Once you have cooked soups and stews, refrigerate them and once they are cold, remove the layer of fat on top.

Snack and Desserts on a Renal Diet

To increase the variety in your diet and make sure you are getting all the calories you need, you might need to add in snacks to your routine. You can add snacks everyday as long as you are at a normal weight or need to gain weight. Be cautious with snacks if you are overweight or your diabetes is not well controlled.

Low Protein Snacks

Fruit: Apples, applesauce, grapes, fruit cocktail, canned pears, pineapple or tangerines

Vegetables: 1/2 cup—1 serving; coleslaw, cucumber, onion, salad, baby carrots, and celery sticks

Starches: low sodium or unsalted crackers, pretzels, popcorn, rice cakes, 1/2 English muffin or bagel

High Protein Snacks

If you are on dialysis, you need additional protein to improve or maintain your nutritional status. Snacks can help you before or after dialysis to get enough calories and protein. Some examples are:

Meat Sandwiches (1/2 or whole)

Low Salt cottage cheese and fruit or low sodium crackers

Chicken or Tuna Salad with crackers

Deviled or Hard Boiled Eggs

Pudding or custard made with non dairy creamer, almond, or rice milk

Healthy Eating For Chronic Kidney Disease
Snack and Desserts on a Renal Diet, cont.

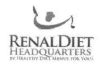

Other options for snacks are below:

- 1.5 ounce pound cake
- Cookies—butter cookies (3), gingersnaps (3 small), 2 ladyfingers, shortbread (2 small), snicker doodle (1), sugar (2)
- 7-8 Vanilla wafers
- 1 3 in square rice crispy bar, homemade
- 8 small sugar wafers
- 1 ounce Teddy Grahams
- 1/4 cup sherbet
- 4 ounce diet lemon lime, ginger ale, or root beer
- 1 slice of white bread
- 3/4 cup rice or corn cereals, unsweetened
- 5 crackers with unsalted tops
- 1 ounce animal crackers
- 3 graham cracker squares
- 2 1/2 cup popcorn, unsalted
- 1 small fresh apple, plum or pear
- 3/4 cup fresh blueberries, pineapple, or 1 cup raspberries
- 1/2 cup fresh or frozen grapes
- 1/2 cup unsweetened applesauce
- 1/2 cup rice milk, unfortified
- 2 rice cakes, any kind
- 1/2 toasted bagel (plain, egg, or cinnamon)
- 1/2 English muffin
- 1/4 cup egg or chicken salad on 5 crackers

Treatment for Low Blood Sugar with CKD

If you are a diabetic and have CKD, you probably already know that hypoglycemia is when your blood sugar level is too low. This can happen because the medications you take cause your blood sugar levels to decrease, and sometimes they get too low. Normal blood sugar levels are between 80—130 mg/dl. Hypoglycemia can occur when your levels are 70 mg/dl or lower.

Symptoms of Hypoglycemia—start with the mild symptoms and moves to the severe if not treated. Sometimes if hypoglycemia occurs during sleep, the person may wake up with the severe symptoms.

Mild Hypoglycemia Symptoms

- Shakiness
- Sweating
- Blurred vision
- Dizziness/lightheadedness
- Anxiety/worry
- Weakness/tiredness
- Headache
- Hunger
- Poor concentration
- Nausea
- Rapid heartbeat

Severe Hypoglycemia Symptoms

- Confusion
- Argumentative/combative
- Extreme Tiredness / weakness
- Seizures / convulsions
- Unconsciousness

Causes of Hypoglycemia

- Taking too much insulin or diabetes medication
- Delaying or skipping a regularly scheduled meal or snack
- Not eating your usual meal or snack before or after your hemodialysis treatment
- Not eating enough carbohydrate at your meal or snack
- Exercising longer or harder than usual
- Drinking alcohol without food

Steps to take if you suspect hypoglycemia

1. If you have a glucometer, check your blood sugar level. If it is below 70 mg/dl then do the following steps. If it is below 40, or the person is exhibiting signs of severe hypoglycemia, call an ambulance as well as doing the steps below.

2. Eat or drink 15 grams of carbohydrate.

    - 3 glucose tablets or a tube of glucose gel
    - 1 Tablespoon of sugar or 3 teaspoons of sugar
    - 6 pieces of regular hard candy (not sugar free)
    - 4 ounces of grape, apple, or cranberry juice
    - 1/2 cup regular lemonade, lemon lime soda, or ginger ale

Treatment for Low Blood Sugar with CKD

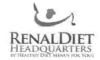

3. Wait about 15 minutes after to allow the food to get into your bloodstream and start raising your levels.

4. Check the blood sugar level again. If your levels have not risen above 70 mg/dl, repeat the first 2 steps.

5. If your blood sugar still has not reached 70 mg/dl or higher after checking three times, then call 911.

6. If you are unable to check your blood sugar level, eat or drink 15 grams of carbohydrate as outlined above and observe behavior to prevent severe low blood sugar.

7. After successful treatment, be sure to eat a snack or meal within one hour to prevent blood sugar dropping too low again.

8. Avoid drinking orange, prune, or vegetable juices since they can be high in potassium. Avoid chocolate candy because they will not give the increase in blood sugar and they contain potassium and phosphorus.

Preventing Hypoglycemia

Avoiding hypoglycemia (low blood sugar) is always better than trying to treat it. Some suggestions to help you avoid hypoglycemia are:

- Take the correct dose of medication for diabetes—use a pill box weekly to lay out your pills or make sure your needles are the same volume to avoid taking too much
- Check blood sugar levels if you exercise—both before and after
- Don't drink alcohol on an empty stomach
- Try to eat your meals and snacks at the same time each day and eat a constant amount of carbohydrate with each meal. Carbohydrate is what makes your blood sugar high if you eat too much.
- If you travel, eat at your normal home times for meals and snacks
- Make sure you always have a quick acting sugar with you like sugar packets, glucose tablets, hard candy, or glucose gel.

Managing Fluid Intake with Dialysis

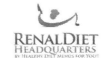

On dialysis, tracking your fluid intake is just as important as what you eat. Your kidneys remove extra fluid from your body, and when they stop working and you are on dialysis, the machine now removes your extra fluid. If you gain too much fluid weight between treatments, you might feel the symptoms listed below. Fluid gains of 5% or more of your body weight increase your risk of heart damage and death. Limiting your fluid as instructed by your nephrologist helps you to feel better between treatments.

Symptoms of Fluid Build-Up

- Shortness of breath
- Dizziness
- Nausea
- Headaches
- Cramping
- High Blood Pressure
- Damage to your heart
- Swelling (esp. around your legs and ankles)

When on dialysis, you need to track and limit your daily fluid intake at mealtimes and between meals, especially if you do not make urine.

Write down how much fluid you take in to keep track until you are able to understand how much to take in consistently.

If you make a small amount of urine—drink or eat no more than 48 ounces per day. (6 cups)

If you do not make urine—drink or eat no more than 32 ounces (4 cups) of fluid each day

To feel your best, try not to gain more than 4—6 pounds between treatments—including weekends.

Food Items that are considered Fluids (Foods that are liquid at room temperature are considered fluids)

- Water
- Milk and Milk Substitutes
- Juices
- Coffee and tea
- Soft drinks
- Alcoholic beverages
- Soups and broths
- Nutritional liquid supplements
- Yogurt
- Pudding
- Custard
- Gelatin
- Smoothies
- Ice chips and cubes
- Popsicles
- Ices and snow cones
- Ice cream, frozen yogurt, and sherbet

Measuring Fluids

Use a measuring cup and pour the fluid into your most used cups and see how many ounces they contain. Typical portions are:

1 mug = 6 ounces = 3/4 cup

1 cup = 8 ounces

1 pint = 16 fluid ounces = 2 cups

1 quart = 32 fluid ounces = 4 cups

Food	Portion	Fluid Volume
Gelatin	1/2 cup	4 fluid ounces
Pudding/Custard	1/2 cup	3 fluid ounces
Popsicle	1 twin bar	3 fluid ounces
Ice Cream	1/2 cup	2.5 fluid ounces
Frozen Yogurt	1/2 cup	3 fluid ounces
Yogurt	1/2 cup	3.5 fluid ounces

Treatment for Low Blood Sugar with CKD

Ways To Control Your Thirst

Do these things to keep from increasing your thirst while you are trying to limit fluid intake

- Avoid salty or spicy foods that tend to increase your thirst
- Chew sugar free gum to increase saliva
- Suck on sugar free hard candy (limited amounts)
- Freeze grapes, strawberries, pineapple, blueberries, or peaches to suck on
- When you do drink, drink ice water instead of sodas to quench your thirst
- Take meds with mealtime liquids instead of between meals when possible.
- Use a room humidifier to moisten the air you breathe.
- If you have diabetes, control it better to keep your blood sugar levels between 80—130 to keep from increased thirst associated with high blood sugar levels.

Final Suggestions

When you limit fluid intake, you help your health and make dialysis easier because:

- You will have less swelling in your legs and ankles
- Your blood pressure will be easier to control
- You will find it easier to breathe, especially when lying down
- You will not be as thirsty when you finish your dialysis treatments
- Your dialysis treatments will be more comfortable and you will have less muscle cramping
- You will have more energy after dialysis treatments
- You will reduce stress on your health and lessen your risk of death

Made in the USA
Columbia, SC
05 November 2017